101 PA School Admissions Essays

Stories of life in the pursuit of medicine

Stephen Pasquini PA-C
with commentaries by Sue
Edmondson

thepalife.com

The PA Life, LLC
Santa Cruz, CA
www.thepalife.com

101 PA School Admissions Essays / Stephen Pasquini PA-C
and Sue Edmondson. -- 1st ed.
ISBN 978-1542446365

This book of essays is dedicated to every pre-PA who aspires to make the world a better place, whose creativity never ceases to amaze, who remind me daily why I am so lucky to be part of this amazing profession; to my patients who teach me the true meaning of perseverance in the face of life's challenges, and to Sue Edmondson whose words of wisdom grace this book and who gives so generously of her time to help others realize their dreams. Finally, to my amazing family and the many readers of the PA Life blog who fill my life with joy beyond words, Thank you!

Contents

Foreword

The curse of the blinking curser

Meet Kate.

Kate hopes to start PA school next year.

She meets all the GPA qualifications for admission into a good school, completed all the prerequisite coursework, has plenty of healthcare experience hours, shadowed a couple PAs, did pretty well on her first pass at the GRE, and she's ready to start putting together her applications.

Nervous, she sits down, opens her laptop, logs into her CASPA account and is confronted with these eleven words:

"Please explain why you are interested in being a physician assistant."

Staring at the blank screen and blinking curser, she tries to think of a way to start her personal statement.

Two hours later, she's still staring at a blank screen.

Kate has spent most of her education writing about things other than herself.

Now she must turn the spotlight inward and explain to an Admissions Committee why she'd be an awesome addition to their program.

1

Kate feels that PA school is the right path for her. But she doesn't know how to explain that feeling to other people.

On top of that, she knows that to be accepted to her top-choice PA school, she must stand out from the hundreds (maybe even thousands) of applicants just like her, vying for the same spot.

So, if she can't explain how she both fits in and stands out, she might not get into PA school at all.

Maybe you relate to Kate's story?

Maybe you're going through the same thing right now?

You have 2.5 Minutes

The average person's reading speed is about 250 words per minute.

The CASPA personal statement allows a 5,000-character and space count (about 625 words).

Therefore, a full-length statement would take an average of 2.5 minutes to read.

You have a very short time in which to make a big impression.

Are you worthy of consideration?

With the average PA school receiving anywhere from 500-1000 applications per year, Admissions Committees are tasked with making difficult decisions between academically similar applicants, using only the application materials presented to them.

I applied to PA school in 2001 before there was a centralized application service.

The disadvantage was that each application was extremely labor intensive. The advantage was that each application was unique to the school and provided an opportunity to differentiate yourself from your peers.

Centralized application services such as the Central Application Service for Physician Assistants (CAPSA), standardized the presentation of information such as grade point averages, GRE scores, transcripts, employment experience and extracurricular activities.

This standardized process makes it difficult for you to differentiate yourself from your peers.

The personal statement will be the instrument that allows you to elaborate on personal characteristics and attributes, and demonstrate to the Admissions Committee that you are worthy of consideration.

What should you write about?

When researchers from the Physician Assistant Education Association (PAEA) performed a computer assisted retrospective analysis of PA personal statements, they found a remarkable similarity in theme content among all statements submitted.

They identified eight major themes mentioned in more than 70% of the statements that were analyzed.

Here they are from most common to least common:

1. experience

2. altruism and the desire to help people

3. role models

4. challenges and hardships

5. personal characteristics

6. positive perception of PA career attributes

7. key accomplishments

8. religious or spiritual quest

When Admissions staff were asked to rate the importance of the previously identified theme content areas, *they ranked work experience and attributes of a PA career as almost equal in importance.*

Hardships the applicant experienced also ranked high in importance, as did the demonstration of empathy.

Least important was ethnicity or socioeconomic status and experience with illness or injury.

Not so personal, personal statements

When questioned, more than two-thirds of PA school administrators have concerns that the personal statement is not an original work by the applicant.

This is not surprising, since a Google search using the term "personal statement" yielded more than 10 million hits, with the first response being a paid advertisement for a company that will prepare your personal statement for you.

And yes, it is true, among these search results is an essay revision service provided by yours truly. But be clear about one thing — we do not prepare your personal statement for you.

Administrators were also concerned that "personal statements do not demonstrate unique or exceptional qualities of the applicants, and that statements exhibit homogeneity of content."

In other words, after a while all the essays started to sound the same.

Why?

Because, applicants are under the impression that the personal statement must conform to certain criteria to be successful.

Surprisingly, despite administrator concerns over homogeneity of content in the CASPA statements, Admissions staff indicated that the most commonly included content was indeed very important in deciding whom to invite for an interview.

The lesson here is to include the important content, only not in a boring way!

101 PA school essays

In this book, we have compiled over 101 actual essay submissions from PA school applicants just like yourself.

We present them to you in their "naked," unedited form.

They run the gamut from mediocre to marvelous. We've added comments and detailed analysis based on information gathered from interviews with Admissions faculty from across the country, and backed by years of professional writing experience.

We show you what works and what doesn't.

This book sheds light on the mystery of a great personal statement.

Whether you want to avoid over-used themes and common grammar errors, or find inspiration for ways to tell your story, it's all here.

How this book can help: Stealing like Picasso

"Good artists copy, great artists steal" ~ *Pablo Picasso*

You probably think of Picasso as a champion of originality, right?

He helped create the contemporary collage. He was one of the leaders of the Cubist movement. He invented constructed sculpture.

But the truth?

He snatched success formulas from other painters.

For instance:

He used a scene from Las Meninas, a 17th century painting by Diego Velázquez, and created 44 new paintings based on that scene.

He copied the central figure in that painting: five-year old Margaret Theresa, the favorite daughter of King Philip IV.

He imitated the painting's arrangements: the maids of honor, the dwarfs, and the reflection of the king and queen are all snatched from the Velázquez painting.

He even re-painted the large dog.

Does anyone think Picasso committed plagiarism?

I don't think so, or why would his 44 paintings all hang in the Picasso Museum in Barcelona?

Picasso didn't plagiarize, because he didn't outright copy. He added his personal touch and his own style to create new paintings — his interpretations of the same scene.

And that is the secret to success.

If you want to write an amazing personal statement you must study the masters and steal their blueprints for success.

Your life in the pursuit of medicine

"There may never be anything new to say, but there is always a new way to say it" ~ Flannery O'Connor

What do you want to write about? A medical trip to Uganda working in a children's orphanage, caring for your dying mom as she received chemotherapy for stage four breast cancer, your own personal health struggle? Whatever it is, it has been said before. Your challenge is to find a new way to say an old thing.

For that, you need your wonderful voice and those unique details that could come only from a frontier where no one else has been — your life.

The subtitle of this book is, "Stories of life in the pursuit of medicine." I encourage you to digest this book as a series of short stories. Place yourself in the shoes of the PA school Admissions Committee.

What captures your attention?

Which applicant essays resonate with you personally?

Which essays have you yearning for more?

The personal statement is more than just an annoying speed bump on your way to PA school — it is an incredible opportunity. It is the summary of your life up to this point, it's about *who* you want to be, *why* you want to be that person and *how* you want to be for years to come.

As you read through these 101 essays, your job isn't so much learning what to write (or not to write), but to discover a place of vulnerability from which to express your thoughts.

It's about sharing the ideas inside your head with other people. Words are just the medium through which this happens.

After reading through the essays in this book, you might be tempted to feel like there's nothing else to say. You may wonder how you're going to write an original essay that will captivate the admissions committee.

I've been there, and you know what?

It's nonsense.

Write as if no one in the world will ever read it.

Say exactly what you feel. Don't think. Just get your thoughts out there in all their disheveled, chaotic glory.

"Steal a bit, "like Picasso.

Then go back and edit.

The formula for the "perfect" essay

You want the formula for writing the perfect essay?

Here it is:

Make sure to answer the question.

It may seem obvious, but many people fail to do this. Your statement needs to address these two important points: your reason(s) for wanting to pursue medicine specifically as a PA and your appeal as a candidate for PA school. If you don't, you will likely (quickly) lose the interest of Admissions Committees.

If it feels inauthentic, it is.

Don't choose a subject matter simply because you think it will impress. Admissions officers prefer to read a much more personal story of learning and growth.

Stop writing from a place of fear.

Believe it or not, this is your time to be creative. If your personal statement makes them laugh, cry, or think, "Aha, this is a person

I'd like to meet," it's more likely the one they'll remember. They will fight for you because they feel a personal attachment.

Address the elephant in the room.

DON'T gloss over any potential red flags. If you have something on your record you think may raise questions when admissions committees review your files — a difficult semester, low science grades, or a gap in your educational history — it's important to use the personal statement as an avenue to address these issues.

The upside to this is that the personal statement is your chance to describe what lessons you learned from what happened. Sometimes applicants who have been through unfortunate circumstances may be inclined to justify or defend what happened. Keep in mind that acknowledging mistakes and highlighting what you learned from them can have a profound effect on even otherwise marginal applications.

Give examples.

It's okay to make an assertion, but follow it up with the proof. When you tell me you are hardworking and compassionate, tell me how you know — perhaps you were the first of your family to go to college, you supported yourself financially for five years and you spent your weekends helping at the winter warming shelter.

Spell the name of the profession correctly.

This happens so often (as you will see throughout this book) and is such an application killer that it is worth mentioning here. The correct name is "physician assistant," not "physician's assistant."

If plural, it is "physician assistants," or if using the acronym, it is

"PAs." If used in the possessive it is "physician assistant's." or if using the acronym, "PA's."

Examples of correct usage:

"The physician assistant's demeanor was warm and welcoming." (possessive)

"The PA's demeanor was warm and welcoming." (possessive)

"The physician assistants I shadowed were warm and welcoming." (plural)

"The PAs I shadowed were warm and welcoming." (plural)

Don't capitalize physician assistant unless it's part of a formal name such as Physician Assistant Greg Jones. Also, anytime you're citing a specific program name or degree title, you'll capitalize the words. For example, it's "Rutgers University Physician Assistant Program," and "Master of Physician Assistant Studies."

Most professions are not capitalized. That includes physician, doctor, nurse, nurse practitioner and dietitian to name a few. Look it up before you use it.

Whatever you do, double-check all your application info to make sure you have it correct everywhere!

Don't give up.

If you have reached a tough patch you might feel like, "Well, I'm just a screw-up. I might as well quit." But you shouldn't. Here's why — we're all screw-ups at some point or another. Take a deep breath and a break, then get back to work.

101 PA School Admissions Essays

Please explain why you are interested in being a physician assistant

<u>Author note</u>: The essays in this book appear as they were submitted in their original, unedited form. You should notice spelling and grammar errors throughout many of them. We left errors in as they are very common mistakes, ones you will want to avoid. We recommend highlighting errors as you encounter them to help you as you write, edit and revise your personal statement.

Essay 1

Why are you here? The question is one I constantly receive from hospital coworkers after mentioning I just graduated from college. As a nurse technician in the intensive care unit, I witness a variety of health complications. But the compassion and care I see constantly from the physician assistants, doctors, and nurses are inspiring. Appreciating their interest, I always respond with a bright smile, stating it's all just a part of my story.

Let's start here: Health and medicine always had a beautiful allure and I couldn't shake my interest in the complicated machine that we call the human body. From reading illustrated human anatomy books in elementary school, to volunteering at the hospital in my hometown throughout high school, the curiosity in medicine never diminished. I found illness and disease a fascinating creation in the biological world. Why are we so susceptible? And how do we fix it? These were and are questions I consistently ask myself. In addition to my interest in the biological world, my general desire to care for those around me fueled my ambition to pursue a career in health care. Volunteering at St. Francis is where I first discovered that I really loved the hospital environment and interacting with the patients and the hospital staff.

Fast forward to college: I want nothing more than to be a health provider and take matters into my own hands to the best of my ability and to make a positive difference in someone's story. Because of this, I want to spread the knowledge that I have accrued about the positive influence a healthy lifestyle has on illness prevention. As an avid runner, my interest in health and wellness serves as motivation to help treat patients all while educating them about the importance of physical health. So I declared my major as a Premedical student, intending to go to medical school.

This changed quickly. Growing up in a military family, I became used to my ability to adapt to unfamiliar environments easily; however, my unexpected freshman year pitfalls became a more powerful learning experience than intended. During that time, I focused heavily on my social life instead of academics, assuming that my high school study habits would suffice for my college level courses. But I soon discovered I was terribly wrong. My concern for my priorities went out the window. I recognized that my personal health, mental wellbeing, and scholarship were greatly suffering because of my lack of care. Unfortunately, by the time I came to that realization, it was too late to turn back. I was disappointed in myself and discouraged about my future, reaching a point where I convinced myself that I wasn't cut out to be in health care.

Seeing my confidence drop and panic set in about my future, my father was actually the one who suggested the physician assistant path to me after several of his military doctor friends told him about profession. My curiosity was sparked and through my research I was thrilled to find that this profession involves everything that I desire in a career – the wonderful opportunity to practice medicine that is challenging and rewarding, the chance to interact with patients thoroughly in a positive way, and the ability to balance work and family. I grew more confident as I realized that pursing a Physician Assistant career was more than perfect for me.

Fueled with newfound perspective and maturity, I challenged myself in the next semester and I came out of my freshman year maintaining the state scholarship that I had worked so hard for in high school, more importantly, I entered into my sophomore year with restored motivation.

The next three years, I was eager about being involved on campus and focusing on school My sophomore year I served on a medical mission team to Nicaragua where I and other students provided healthcare to the underserved. Here I had the opportunity to witness our team physician in action, as he was able to simultaneously soothe nervous patients and all while expertly assessing vital signs. Inspired by my trip to Nicaragua, I soon obtained my nursing aide certification in my hometown in hopes of being able to gain clinical experience during my senior year of college.

Unfortunately, I had difficulty in finding employment as a CNA due to scheduling conflicts but found a great alternative in volunteering at a free clinic in ****** called Mercy Health Center during my senior year. Mercy's sole purpose is to provide exceptional medical care to the low-income people of ******, *******. At Mercy I first witnessed the compassionate care that the handful of physician assistants, doctors, and nurses who volunteered their time late in the evenings after their workdays to provide healthcare to those who are unable to obtain it. Not only did this experience allow me to interact with patients, I had the chance to observe physicians and physician assistants to gain an understanding of working as a medical provider. In addition, my final semester of college I was taking a course that was mentally challenging and was almost convinced that it would cost me my future; however, Mercy provided consolation through that semester, only confirming that being a PA is my future. The smiles from patient's, genuine tears of happiness, and multiple thank you's were enough to keep me strong for the remainder of school.

So now we're here: As a nurse tech in the ICU at ******, I have gained an unexpected amount of patience and understanding. From the nurses, PA's, and doctors, I have learned how to grow more empathetic, caring, and calm. Overall, I try to remind myself of compassion for others that God has graced me with. . .and in the end, my story to writing this statement follows that of what I want for every person and patient that I have the privilege of interacting with. I had a dream. I found myself low, lost and needing help. But through people believing in me and their guidance and teamwork, our hard work, I became well again. That's my story.

The stars are to block the names of locations for private purposes.

Commentary Essay 1

Your essay starts out with an engaging sentence. I immediately want to know more. For a first draft you've got a good start — you include important information about your interest in medicine, some of the skills you've gained, your compassion and the issue of a lower GPA.

However, the essay has some big problems, starting with its length. It's well over the CASPA limit at almost 6000 characters/spaces. Both count, so you have much to cut. You could eliminate most of the second paragraph for example. I'm going to show you how I'd cut it and correct grammar errors while I'm doing it. I'm also getting rid of contractions, which are disfavored in academic essays, even though they're not grammatically incorrect. Watch for descriptions that are distracting, such as "beautiful allure." It stopped me because I had to think what you meant, and that's not what you want your readers to do. Keep it simple.

Here's the edited paragraph: "Let me start here: health and medicine have always had an allure. From reading anatomy books in elementary school, to volunteering at the local hospital throughout high school, my curiosity in medicine never diminished. In addition, my desire to care for those around me fueled my ambition to pursue a career in health care. Volunteering is where I first discovered that I really loved the hospital environment and interacting with the patients and the hospital staff."

You can do the same throughout, and you'll have to do a lot of cutting because you have more to add. There's not enough to specifically about why you want to be a PA. You talk generally about providers and what you admire about them, but that's not what Admissions folks are looking for. They want to know why you've chosen the PA profession — write about what appeals to you about the role of PA, and why it's better for you than a physician or NP, for example. And it's a really, really bad idea to say that you picked the PA profession because you didn't think you could make the cut for medical school. That's what your essays suggests.

Unfortunately, the essay has other problems, too. The second sentence is incomplete, and by the third sentence you're completely off the topic you start with. This is a problem throughout the essay. Each sentence must lead to the next, and each paragraph has to follow the preceding one.

Essay 2

"Are you still there, Kay?" The elderly patient at the physical therapy clinic where I work quickly became panicked if the physical therapist or I moved out of her peripheral vision. "Yes I'm still here. Take your time and keep going, you're doing great," I replied, resting my hand on her back for support as she slowly tried to take another step forward on the treadmill. The patient, who had previously suffered a stroke, tilted her head to look at me and said, "You have excellent bedside manner, Kay. You will make a wonderful PA one day." I would be lying if I didn't say that comments like these make me feel blessed to be coming in contact with different kinds of people every day, gaining healthcare experience that I can use to make a positive impact on their lives. There is nothing more rewarding than learning how to serve others and educate them on how to improve their quality of life. I want to become a physician assistant because I have a passion for problem solving, learning and encouraging everyone I come in contact with. Being a physician assistant is not only a career, but also a lifestyle, as I would not only treat patients, but also educate, uplift, soothe and invest in patients as well as the families of patients.

Every physician assistant I have come in contact with simply reaffirms my desire to become one, as they consistently take their time with each patient, ease any concerns the patient may have and educate each patient on the condition before leaving the room. My current healthcare experience has adequately prepared me for your PA program. I have learned to work on a team with people holding different positions in a clinical setting, as well as being able to exercise autonomy when preparing treatments for different patients. Physical therapists and physicians have trusted me to administer modalities to patients without being supervised and have often called on me to help them work directly with a patient. I thoroughly enjoy being on a team with physicians and physical therapists, working toward the same goal of restoring our patients to full health. However, I long for the opportunity to be able to diagnose, treat, and educate my own patients.

Volunteering in the emergency room at my local hospital has exposed me to many different cultures and conditions I previously had no knowledge of. I feel privileged to have witnessed the different domestic situations I have, for they have given me a better understanding of an underserved community that I simply cannot ignore. I am currently involved in an outreach program at my church, making meals for the homeless and distributing them to needy individuals in Detroit. I am also in the process of applying to volunteer at FernCare, a free clinic in Ferndale, MI whose aim is to provide nonemergency care to the uninsured population in Oakland County. I am looking to become more familiar with the underserved population, as I desire to practice as a physician assistant in an area with a great need for medical care.

While my experience in healthcare has shown me that I have a passion for medicine and for others, my dedication and horsepower in the last two years of school has solidified in my mind that I have the drive and discipline to successfully complete your physician assistant program. Familiar with the routine of taking many credits while working part time, I know how to stay on track and handle the stress that life brings in healthy ways. I have also become somewhat of a leader in my statistics class that I am currently taking. Students in the class feel comfortable asking me to help explain lessons and study with them, because I am willing to collaborate with a group of people and enjoy helping others learn something new.

For me, becoming an excellent physician assistant is my long term goal. I look forward to serving in multiple hospitals and clinics that are in need of physician extenders. I find happiness in being around people, encouraging others and doing everything in my power to help in any way possible. With the increase in aging population, including retiring physicians, the need for physician assistants has never been greater. I dream of becoming a physician assistant to serve in areas that have a great need, which is where the physician assistant occupation was established. To me, there could be nothing more rewarding than committing my life to the cause of bettering someone else's.

Commentary Essay 2

I can see you've spent a lot of time on your essay. Overall, it's well done. Opening with a nervous patient and showing your compassion —resting your hand on her back for support, is great. I'd like to know what your job is though, and I bet I'm not alone. Then you'd want to break up the first paragraph. This sentence, "I want to become a physician assistant because I have a passion for problem solving, learning and encouraging everyone I come in contact with," should be a new paragraph. But I'd like to see a lead-in sentence or two about how you got to this point — why and how you decided to be a PA in the first place. This is a common problem — we know our story and it's in our heads, but doesn't make it to the page.

If the sentence that starts with "Volunteering in the emergency room . . ." isn't already a new paragraph, it needs to be. And I'd move the second sentence of that paragraph, "I feel privileged to have witnessed the different domestic situations I have, for they have given me a better understanding of an underserved community that I simply cannot ignore," down to the second to last sentence of the paragraph. You need transitions between the other sentences in that paragraph, too. They don't flow as well as they should.

I also wouldn't write, "your program." Assuming you're going through CASPA, everyone knows chances are you are targeting more than one program. So, it feels false. One other thing — don't use contractions. They're disfavored in academic essays. Show you know and respect the rules.

Essay 3

I was twenty years old when I first learned what the word death truly meant. Up until that point, I knew that death existed, but I didn't know what it felt like to see a dead body in front of me. The more I think about that day, the more that it angers me. There lay my sweet Sally whom I had grown to love over the past four months, and all my director of nursing could say was how happy she was to finally have a bed free. How could someone I looked up to as a mentor, be so careless when it came to the life of another human being? Why did this person who took a job as a healthcare provider, treat another human life as if it were nothing? In that moment, I knew that my purpose in the medical field was far kinder and greater than that of the person I had looked up to and respected for so long.

Throughout my life, I have used my challenges and shortcomings to motivate me. As a person who aspires to be a physician assistant one day, I know in my heart of hearts that this is what I am meant to do. Am I a hardworking person? Absolutely. Am I a team player who works well with other people? Without a doubt. But, what makes me distinctly qualified to pursue a professional degree as a Physician Assistant at D'Youville College, is my compassion and kindness towards other people. I want this career, not because of money or job security, but because I truly want to make a difference in the lives of people that I touch. I want to be remembered not by my title, but what I did with my title to help people in a positive manner.

Recently, a physician assistant that I work with suggested that I consider a career as a physician assistant. Inspired by her story, I began to dig deeper. Based on interpersonal and internet resources I have concluded that although a registered nurse can treat an acute or long standing illness, they have very little authority in the long-term medical plan of a patient. Although a nurse practitioner can do most things that a physician assistant can do, they are usually limited by licensure to one area of medicine. A physician assistant on the other hand, has the skills needed to treat and prevent a wide range of illnesses, in many aspects of the medical field. More often than not, as a physician assistant, you are developing long-term care plans and personal relationships that g above and beyond that of a twelve-hour shift.

When I think about that day six years ago when I experienced death for the first time, I am reminded of one thing. Death taught me about life. And although I lost all respect for my mentor that day, I learned just how important the idea of humanity is.

Commentary Essay 3

The essay shows your great compassion, which is excellent. And you tie your beginning to the end. Great job there. However, there are a few things that need work.

One is this sentence: "But, what makes me distinctly qualified to pursue a professional degree as a Physician Assistant at D'Youville College, is my compassion and kindness towards other people." I hate to say it, but 99.9% of the people who apply to PA school are kind and compassionate. While these qualities are essential, in my opinion, to a great healthcare provider, they're not unique to PAs, or among PA applicants. So this sentence not only doesn't help you, it detracts because it undermines the reader's belief that you really know what the profession is about.

Since you work with a PA, instead of referring to your research to explain why you want to be a PA (especially Internet research, which is a very weak thing upon which to base a career choice), use your personal experiences to tell explain your decision. What have you witnessed the PA do with patients that you admire? What appeals to you about the work? Don't talk about it in the third person ("you are developing long-term care plans and personal relationships . . ."). Keep it personal to what you like about the profession. You can distinguish the PA's role from others, but do it without talking about the Internet. Also, you might want to explain why you want to be a PA before you get to what is now the second paragraph.

You don't need to slam your mentor in the end, either. End on a positive note. By the way, physician assistant isn't capitalized unless it's part of a formal name, and when you write, "a Physician Assistant at D'Youville College," it shouldn't be capitalized.

Essay 4

I was barely nineteen and up to my ears in feces. I stood in a room where nearly a dozen infants ranging from fifteen to twenty months lived out their days on a large mat at Imani orphanage in Nairobi, Kenya. Diarrhea dribbled over my hand and ran down my threadbare apron, trickling onto my thigh where the edge of the apron bunched up beneath the child resting on my hip. I held her away and ran for fresh diaper cloths, the ones I'd hand washed yesterday in a giant plastic barrel and hung to drip over gravel beneath the hot Kenyan sun.

My best friends were starting their second semesters of college, but I'd chosen to wait and serve. In the months I spent at Imani, I learned more about life and service than during my next four years of college.

Service is messy, not glamorous. It's slow. It's unnoticed. And it's the most profound thing a human being can do for another.

One day, I saw a petite woman of Indian heritage enter the baby room. She was a doctor. Several babies were dying of HIV/AIDS, and at least half of them had a fever on any given day. I listened to her story, watched her work in what seemed like a hopeless situation, and knew where I was called to serve.

I'd always been interested in medicine; always pulling teeth and digging at splinters and reading books on first aid but once I saw the impact a good doctor can have on a person's mind, body, and soul, I was hooked. A commitment to medical service gives others a passport to life. I entered college a year late. Every summer, when my fellow premed students clamored for paper pushing internships at doctor's offices, I hit the streets and worked between eighty and hundred hours a week selling SAT prep and home-work reference books to families, cold calling door to door. It was the only way I could pay for my schooling.

Being one of six children in a family from rural Kentucky, I occasionally sent money home, not vice versa. If serving taught me about life, selling taught me about people, communication, and hard work. The rejection made me stronger, the challenge developed resolve, and the difficulties became blessings in disguise. I'd always had medical school on the back burner, but the seven summers I spent recruiting, training, and managing sales teams revealed to me that I enjoyed building people more than running a business.

While taking blood pressure and patient complaints during a medical trip to Honduras, I learned about the position of a physician assistant from the team's doctor, and the model resonated strongly with how I'm wired. I'm passionate about relationship building, quality time with people, and the flexibility to be a life-long learner by investing time in multiple specialties. I love the idea of empowering doctors to focus on their strengths by shouldering some of their burden. To me, a physician's assistant serves not only her patients, but her doctor, her community, and her world. My application isn't stellar. My path through PA school began just this August when I enrolled in an EMT class. I've taken my time investigating precisely what direction I should choose. But I'm not afraid of rejection: I know how I want to serve. I don't have to travel to a village in Honduras or an orphanage in Kenya to find needy people and underserved areas. It's right here in my own backyard and I'm asking you if you will be willing to instruct me in what it takes to change a community one service at a time.

Commentary Essay 4

First the really bad news — you have an error that would likely keep you from an interview, and that's getting the name of the profession wrong. It is not physician's assistant, ever. It is physician assistant. Okay, now onto the content.

I was captivated by your opening. Great job. In fact, most of the essay was great. When I got here, "I'd always had medical school on the back burner, but the seven summers I spent recruiting, training, and managing sales teams revealed to me that I enjoyed building people more than running a business," I was a bit confused. Not all doctors run businesses if that's your point.

Also, when you say your application isn't stellar, you should expand on that and explain what you mean. Finally, I recommend people not use contractions because they're disfavored in academic essays.

Essay 5

My interest in becoming a physician assistant sparked when I was young watching my mother fight and eventually overcome her many idiopathic gastrointestinal problems. At the time, I only understood that a nice white coated man had earned my mother's trust with his compassion. While her primary physician was quite helpful and knowledgeable, it was the physician assistant (PA) who truly made the difference in my mother's health care and spent the most time with her. He was the first one to see her and walk through her medical history. Her PA was the one to connect with her, get to know her and my family, and come up with the preliminary treatment plan, which he then continuously tweaked in order to alleviate all her symptoms. As a young child, seeing my mother freed from the all-encompassing discomfort that had plagued her for months was astonishing, and her PA left a great impression on me that stayed for many years. At the time, I did not realize that this man was a PA, but the warmth and support of that experience planted a desire to enter the medical world. Acting on this growing curiosity, I began try on different provider hats by caring for my Barbie. Using various instruments such as plastic knives, scotch tape, and screwdrivers, I would fix Barbie's 'broken footitis' and other ailments and triumphantly return her in one piece to Ken. With time, my understanding of the medical field has evolved, and set me on a path to become a PA.

In my senior year of high school, I was privileged to be able to work with a research team from the National Institutes of Health. I shadowed a few of the doctors as they visited their patients and appreciated the complete trust that the patients had for them. I observed that the trust was in part built by the doctors' willingness to explain every aspect of the disease and treatment using comprehensible language. I was impressed by their patience and communication, and that teaching atmosphere influenced me when I became a Red Cross instructor teaching First Aid/CPR/AED for the first responder while in college. I educated students, professors, and locals so I had to find different ways of instructing a diverse crowd. It was then I realized how I enjoyed working with and educating people. That 'oh!' moment as the students understood the concept was incredibly gratifying.

After graduation, I began working at the Johns Hopkins Hospital Adult Emergency Department (ED). There I was able to observe how doctors, nurses, PAs, nursing practitioners, social workers, and many other support staff roles came together to form a cohesive team, and the idea of becoming a PA firmly took root. Witnessing their dedication in treating their patients, I was reminded of my mother's PA from so many years ago. I gained a deeper and more valuable insight into the PA profession after working alongside exceptional PAs for the past three years.

As a HIV counselor in the ED, I have been fortunate to be able to work with a very diverse population with intensely varied needs, behaviors, and backgrounds. It was incredibly challenging at first to counsel patients regarding their risky health and sexual behaviors but I quickly adapted, adjusted my approach, and became much more comfortable in such difficult situations. I was thrilled to be able to work with patients and educate them on how to keep themselves and their partners protected from sexually transmitted diseases and persuade them to practice healthier sexual behaviors. With this position, I truly understood the trust and intimacy patients have with their health care providers as patients not only divulged personal details regarding their sexual life, but sometimes their entire life history as frustrated patients unloaded about how HIV has impacted their lives. With newly diagnosed positive patients, I worked together with their PA to counsel them and establish their next steps. Working behind the scenes coordinating the HIV testing program has also granted me further opportunities to observe them as they consulted me regarding their out of care positive patients and at times, gently persuade the reluctant patient to obtain care.

My respect for PAs only strengthened after shadowing a few. I witnessed as they deftly balanced their independence as a health provider with coordinating with their supervising physicians. As in the case with my mother, the PAs were the one to spend the majority of the time with the patient as well as decide on the treatment. The physicians hold the PAs' decisions in high esteem and rarely change the orders.

All my experiences have coalesced the challenges and rewards of being a PA and have reinforced my resolve to become one. I have seen how important it is to be one of the first lines of communication and how an individual may benefit from compassionate and sensitive health providers. I am eager to further my health training so that I can impact patients' lives the way that I have watched amazing PAs do so again and again, and especially in the way my mother's PA has affected ours.

Commentary Essay 5

Good job on bringing PAs into the essay right up front. Sometimes people don't mention PAs until the essay is nearly over, and I've even seen some that never mention the profession at all.

You could shorten up that first paragraph some, though. Leave out the sentence starting with this: "While her primary physician was quite helpful . . .," and the ones about Barbie and Ken. Your essay is over the character count to begin with, and frankly, those types of childhood stories waste important characters and spaces.

You gloss over your experiences working with PAs. Not many applicants have worked alongside them for three years! Talk about your experiences, and use those to specifically write about why you are choosing the profession. Rather than a generic sentence such as this: "I gained a deeper and more valuable insight into the PA profession after working alongside exceptional PAs for the past three years," be specific about your observations.

Read your sentences carefully. I'm not sure what this means, ". . . they consulted me regarding their out of care positive patients," and while I can guess, I shouldn't have to. The sentence as a whole is long and awkward.

This sentence isn't grammatically correct, "All my experiences have coalesced the challenges and rewards of being a PA . . ." Watch for those things, too.

You want the last sentence of the essay to be very strong, and by ending with this phrase, "especially in the way my mother's PA has affected ours," isn't. You can include that in your conclusion, but not as the last word.

Essay 6

"Your baby's blood sugar levels are below normal on the third day of life. We need to take him to the NICU for further evaluation" said a pediatrician. It has been a year since I had heard those words, but it still feels like it has happened recently. The day I was going to take my newborn son home, his pediatrician was convinced that he needs to stay until his blood sugar levels stabilize. It was devastating to see my son that seemed perfectly healthy to me with wires all over his body that were attached to the monitor. It is hard to explain how you feel to someone who has never been through the similar situation. My son was in NICU for four weeks and that experience have changed my life and my perspective. Devastation, helplessness, guilt, blame, sadness, and hope were the first emotions I experienced. Uncertainty about his diagnosis and his treatment plan for the first two weeks and unknown length of time he would stay there made it more difficult.

However, at this point of my life I am thankful for this personal experience. It was traumatic at the time, but it has helped me in many ways that were unclear earlier. I have learned the difference between poor care and an outstanding care for the patient.

I was inspired to follow my dreams to become a PA by a great doctor and a wonderful caring Physician Assistant. It would be unfair to say that only a PA made a difference. I am sincerely thankful to a group of nurses, endocrinology specialist, and a primary care doctor that were taking care of my son. It was a PA though who took the time to explain and teach us about my child's diagnosis, his treatment plan, and the best management of his condition. It was a PA who would ask me what I could suggest or consider, who would notice that I was hesitant about some decisions made by the doctor. He would go out of his way to discuss any possibilities with the doctors and consult other specialists regarding our case. I received an invaluable experience about the importance of patients' feelings, sincere care, and an ability to accept that there are always ways to expand and research on any condition or treatment plans. Commitment to Volunteering at Ronald Mc Donald House will be an opportunity for me to thank those who saved my child's life through helping others.

A further experience with shadowing a PA in pediatric orthopedic surgery was another great way to learn a difference between an outstanding health care and a poor health care. I do not believe in average care because one cannot help just fifty percent out of a hundred. If a person makes a decision to help saving people's lives, to treat their health problems, then he/she takes a responsibility to provide the best possible care that will most likely change someone's life. It has to be an exceptional service and less than "best" is simply unacceptable. The PA I am still shadowing have taught me that compassion towards patients, nonjudgmental approach, and consideration of their personal choices can be well balanced with a knowledgeable and professional treatment. Since she has to communicate with children and their parents she takes the time to explain the details of the treatment and answer the questions in a manner that would be satisfactory and clear to both. Her humble attitude, her desire to learn more from her colleagues and attending doctors, her ability to be a team player and initiate willingness to help in a variety of hospital settings show a great example of a PA I want to be. I have learned plenty of technical terms and treatment plans from her. But the paramount knowledge that I obtained consists of a devotion to the selfless service to others.

I admit that working as a medical assistant, as an acupuncturist, and a medical office manager helped me to understand a healthcare, a role of different medical providers, hands-on patient experience, and identify a path that I want to take. However, those experiences that made me fall and get up again, unexpected life threat to my child, and the patients that had no hope for recovery gave me the strength and true understanding of the profession I chose. I believe that my healed bruises are the most valuable steps in becoming an exceptional healthcare provider and the best PA I can be.

Commentary Essay 6

I'm was very sorry to read that you and your baby had to go through such a traumatic experience. It speaks volumes about your character that you found a positive in the experience. It's a good way to open your essay. We are engaged because it's about you and your baby.

However, what happens is that you lose me because of the grammar. It starts with a small error — you leave out the comma here: evaluation" said a pediatrician. It should be evaluation," said the pediatrician. (Note, I've changed it to "the" pediatrician, because it's not just any old one — it's the one treating your child). Next you combine present and past tense: "his pediatrician was convinced that he needs to stay." It should read "needed" to stay. Next comes this: "experience have changed," which should be "experience has changed."

Grammar matters to Admissions folks as they told me when I interviewed them for our book, "How To Write Your Physician Assistant Personal Statement." All said there shouldn't be any grammar errors, that it was a red flag that people didn't pay attention to details. In healthcare, missing the details can lead to death! There are other grammar problems throughout. It will be your job to spot them since this isn't a formal edit.

I wouldn't make your main point good care versus bad care. That can apply to any health care profession. Focus on something PA related when you get to the shadowing experience. And when you talk about the team that helped you and your child, rather than saying: "It would be unfair to say that only a PA made a difference," focus on how the PA's role complemented that of the physician and other team members.

Essay 7

"Felicitaciones está embarazada", I said with a smile to Maria, as she sat across from a Panamanian doctor and me; Maria's two young children were below her playing on the dirt floor of the old school house turned doctor's office. With tears in her eyes and a large smile accompanying, she reached across the table and hugged me. The joy she emitted at the news of her pregnancy filled room and at that moment something changed in me for I knew that I was on the right path towards becoming a Physician Assistant.

As an undergrad I had the opportunity to spend part of my summer in rural Panama as a member of a medical brigade. In

Panama I witnessed the lack of accessible medical care, which made me appreciate the healthcare accessibility we have as Americans. Every day, to my amazement, several hundred people had gathered from surrounding villages to receive medical attention. The experiences I had throughout this mission developed a passion to medically serve in an underserved community. I want to make a difference in my future community by providing better access to care and to develop long-term genuine relationships with my patients.

My admiration for the PA profession grew during my time shadowing. The PA's I followed were autonomous, efficient, and attentive when consulting patients. During my time of shadowing I observed PA's briefly expressing concerns or clarifying ideas with a physician every few hours. This insight into the PAMD relationship demonstrates that there must be an immense amount of trust and teamwork in order to deliver excellent healthcare to patients. Shadowing truly opened my eyes to the importance a PA is to a medical practice and its patients.

Working as a physical therapy aide has given me valuable experience in conversing and treating a wide range of patients in a one to one setting. At the clinic in which I work there is one physical therapist and two aides. As a PT aide I have seen patients with a diverse range of ages, injuries, personalities, and ethnicities. Patients are treated for over an hour, which allows us to truly know them throughout their weeks or even years in therapy. My time here has taught me that healthcare is more than just a service. It requires a holistic understanding of a patient's life and history as well as their specific medical issue. Some patients have issues that are deeper than their current injury or condition and it is part of a good medical professional's duty to understand these nuances as they become familiar with their patients. I have noticed the physical therapist may take on several roles when treating patients. Some roles are motherly, some are motivational, and with some patients she must show a gentle yet firm authority in order to execute effective treatments. Having the privilege to work closely with someone who cares so much about her patients has provided me a great starting point for the rest of my career.

Like the PAMD relationship, a PT aide must also work closely with the Physical Therapist. The PT must have trust in the aide to achieve the specific treatment plan for each patient. A PA may go about their day visiting their scheduled patients with little supervision from the MD, just as a PT aide must listen to, instruct, and care for patients with little supervision in a physical therapy setting.

With an educational background in physiology and a life of sports and exercise, I decided to try my hand at personal training last summer. One client – now friend Lisa, said I saved her life. Over a summer of training she lost 20% of her body weight and to this day we stay in contact even though I no longer work as a trainer. She sends me photos of her rock climbing, skiing, and doing things she claims she would have never done if it weren't for me. The pride this gives me I liken to that of a parent watching their child graduate college. Having the taste of someone's pure happiness and healthy living as a result of coming to me with their troubles is extremely rewarding. I would be privileged to pursue my passion in medicine and the satisfaction in the betterment of peoples' lives for the remainder of my life as a PA.

Over the last several years of volunteering in multiple Seattle hospitals I have observed PA's in several settings. Their quick critical thinking skills and ability to swiftly develop of a plan of action with the physician are attributes I believe I will excel at.

A career in healthcare is not for the weak of heart and I understand the long hours, meticulous charting, emotional strains, as well as the potential changes and adaptations in healthcare. My experiences have confirmed that I am made for this career and cannot wait to travel upon the strenuous yet rewarding path towards becoming a Physician Assistant.

Commentary Essay 7

First the technical items — physician assistant isn't capitalized unless it's part of a formal name, such as Brown School of Physician Assistant Studies. You also make a very common grammar error — using the singular of a noun (PA) and plural (their) in the same sentence. It's a problem in more than one place in the essay. Even though it's common, there's no reason to make it. As you'll see me say time and again, those mistakes matter to Admissions folks. They expect grammar-error free essays.

As to content, it's excellent. You did a great job of bringing the reasons you want to be a PA to life. The one thing I would change is switching the second to last paragraph with the one that precedes it.

Essay 8

"Will you be taking out the stitches?" The doctor looked at me questioningly, but before I translated into English what our Hispanic patient had said, I took a second to appreciate what she was asking. I was just there to shadow in the minor surgery clinic that day, but ended up filling in as an interpreter. Throughout the lumpectomy, I had been holding the patient's hand and reassuring her. I did not touch a medical instrument. Yet this patient trusted me to be the one to remove her sutures when she returned the next week, because I was there for her through a touch and a language she could understand. I knew then that patient care was the right place for me.

Though my path to this point was not a direct one, it allowed me to take advantage of diverse opportunities, all of which I can draw on as a future physician assistant.

If I had known I wanted to study medicine, I would not have taken art as an elective throughout high school. Instead I would have focused on science coursework, and missed learning something that cannot be found in a textbook. While painting, I learned to look at the piece as a whole. When one is concentrating on a portion of the work, they still must step back and see how the whole piece is affected. That one suspicious lump on her breast did not define my patient. She is a whole person: within a culture and community, with fears and hopes. As a PA, I will view the disease in light of the person. Aside from their clinical cases, patients' cultures may differ, impacting not only how they understand their illness but also how they are willing to treat it. My goal will not only be to come to the correct diagnosis but to find a way to effectively communicate that diagnosis with the patient, answering their questions and empowering them in their healthcare.

If I had known I wanted to study medicine, I might not have spent a semester abroad in Ecuador. I would never have volunteered in a women's prison daycare, where infants who spend the night in their mother's cell are cared for by day. Some of the caregivers' methods were the opposite of what my Child Development classes had taught me, such as routinely striking the children. At times it was frustrating and hard to keep volunteering, yet I knew that trying to explain Erikson's theories or change how their culture raises children was not the answer. While I stayed true to my beliefs, I realized that we all wanted the best for these kids, to prepare them to enter the world and succeed. Our cultures taught us different directions, but we were journeying toward the same place and cooperation was key. Through this experience I learned that being a member of a healthcare team means working together, despite differences of opinion. Though the team is made up of individuals, we have a common goal: to improve the health and wellbeing of our patients and their families.

Now I know I want to be a physician assistant – a profession where teamwork is built in. In my current job as a clinic assistant at California Sports and Orthopedic Institute, I have not only built relationships with the doctors and PAs that I work with but also with the patients. I am already part of a healthcare team. I converse with patients, remove their sutures, and reassure them as I prepare a scheduled injection. I pull up relevant scans for the providers and obtain insurance authorizations to help them continue to care for their patients. In addition to my post baccalaureate studies and full time job, I founded a group for other pre-PA students. We share ideas and experiences. I have reached out to PAs that I know and organized events where they came and answered our questions. Patients will not be successfully treated if their healthcare providers are in competition to prove they are right; we should always be helping each other succeed.

I am motivated to learn in any way I can. When I have time, I read the doctors' dictations and write down any term or condition I do not know to look up or ask our PA, Gaye, about later. While taking anatomy I would ask Will, our x-ray technician, to pull up different scans so I could try to identify bony landmarks on a real person. Occasionally I wake up at 5 am to go on hospital rounds with Gaye even though I do not start work until 8:30. I observe surgery and practice suturing with a string tied to my desk at home. I will endeavor to learn something new from each patient I treat. Each will have a story, making the experience more memorable and powerful. I will never stop learning or pushing myself to be the best physician assistant I can be. I am excited to start that journey now.

Commentary Essay 8

This is a very clever essay and very well done. It is a bit risky because you really don't specify why you want to be a PA, but it's certainly implied. You could slip in a few specifics in that second to last paragraph, cleverly, as you've written the rest of the essay.

Essay 9

Terrified and afraid, I stood at the door of the hospital room where my mother was. I was so shaken by the consequence of the accident everything seemed illusory. It was hard to see my mother on the hospital bed smiling at me, trying to give me strength. That hot day in August, my mother lost her right arm in a bus accident, I can clearly remember the doctors going in and out of her room, I too afraid to enter, stood at the door. Life as I knew changed forever. For the past 18 years my mother has learned to become independent and do everything on her own, while raising 6 children. She is my motivation, the reason I always pushed myself to overcome my fears and continue towards my dreams. With over 1000 hours of healthcare experience working in a collaborative setting, my personality endorsed the ability to interact with others and understand the difficulties that people face, preparing me to follow the Physician Assistant path.

Since high school, I had developed a strong interest in the biological sciences. I participated in the Science Research Program and became the first student from my high school to be accepted into the Rockefeller University Outreach Program. For the next two years, I conducted reached at the Vosshall Lab assisting Fellow Graduates with their research. In order to afford the expense of traveling to the city I obtained a job at a local supermarket.

I truly became in love with the medical field during my summer trips to Pakistan. While visiting family and trying to understand my background I was able to appreciate the countless opportunities that I was presented with in the US. Being a first generation Immigrant I was able to recognize that life presents people with many hardships and it is what we make of it. Seeing people in immediate need, I developed resilient feelings lead to the realization that I wanted to be in a profession where I would be able to feel good about what I do on a daily basis.

I love the feeling of fulfillment when you know you have made a difference for someone. I was able to achieve that emotion while working as a Resident Services Assistant and Resident Medication Assistant at a Senior Assisted living. While providing assistance with daily activities, care and administering medications I was able to connect and develop a friendly relationship with the residents. Most of the residents are dealing with numerous difficulties, some having lost a spouse after 60 years of marriage, or trying to understand Parkinson's Syndrome. One day I walked into one of the resident, Sarah's room to check on her and found her on the floor, her face covered in blood, conscious, she looked at me and said, "I don't know what happened". I immediately called 911 and stayed to comfort her; this showed I could be both empathetic and emotionally resilient in the face of calamity. Over the months I was faced with situations where I had to send out the residents via 911. As a Med tech, I became familiar with not only medications but also the dosages and the side effects. Through my job I was able to develop analytical, incident response, and risk analysis skills that will surely benefit me tremendously as a PA.

My immense familiarity with the geriatrics population and pediatrics, from volunteering at Sunshine Children's home and Rehab center, has expanded my knowledge. With the Valley Hospital PA Shadowing Program, I was able to acquaint myself with the responsibilities of PA in vast specialties including Breast oncology, Weight loss surgery and Internal Medicine. I am completely fascinated by the trusting relationship between the physician and the PA. By the end of May, I will have over 200 hours of shadowing experience. From my professional involvements I can say with confidence that I would be a trustworthy PA with a pliable scope of practice, rather than be tied down to a single specialty.

Being a PA will allow me to exemplify my care for humanity and assist in using my knowledge to help others and also be able to provide a great lifestyle for my family. The PA field requires not only hard work and compassion but also dedication and commitment. Through my personal and professional experiences, I believe I have the personality to succeed as a PA. Knowing that my expertise can make someone's life better motivates me to make my dream come true.

Commentary Essay 9

Wow, what a story about your mom. It's definitely compelling, but would be even more compelling (as would the rest of the essay) without the distraction of overly descriptive adjectives and verbs, often used in the wrong way.

Now, as a first generation immigrant (which by the way, should not be capitalized), perhaps English is not your first language and that's part of the reason. However, you're not alone — incorrect use of adjectives and verbs is a common issue I see among applicants. Regardless, less is more. So use plain words instead of writing such as this: "... my personality endorsed the ability ...," or "...with a pliable scope of practice ..." and "I developed resilient feelings lead ..." Apart from the odd use of "pliable," you left out "that" and misspelled "led." Misspelling "led" is a universal mistake that I see in countless essays. "Lead" is present tense and "led" is past tense.

Also, a couple of grammar points — don't capitalize physician assistant unless it's part of a formal name or you're applying to a specific school that capitalizes it, spell out numbers one through nine except when telling time or in ages, the end punctuation always goes outside the quotation marks. And watch for missing commas.

Every sentence in these short essays must count. Unless there's a PA-related reason to include the sentence about working in a supermarket, such as it introduced you to diverse cultures, out it goes. By the way, you missed a comma after "city."

Essay 10

I have always known that I wanted to have a job in the medical field. From very early on I was interested in the sciences and medicine. Throughout high school Anatomy and Physiology was the class I couldn't wait to go to and when it was over I didn't want to leave. Midway through college I had an experience that really solidified my decision. I was sitting on the couch with my boyfriend and some of his friends one day when he suddenly began to seize violently. I immediately knew what was happening and tried to get him on his side. One of his friends dialed 911 while we moved the furniture away from him so he wouldn't injure himself. I have a true calling to medicine, and especially becoming a physician assistant.

I first learned about the physician assistant profession when I began researching careers in the medical field during my freshman year of college. There were so many positives about the PA profession that I was instantly interested. Not only could I diagnose and treat patients, but I could also change specialties if I ever decided to. Also, by working as a team with a doctor, tough diagnoses could be discussed to give the patient the best form of treatment. While shadowing at Faith Family Medical, I really saw the positive relationships between nurse practitioners, PA's, and physicians. They would perform their daily duties independently, but if a question arose, there was no hesitation to ask others for advice. After shadowing a PA and working in a healthcare environment, the PA profession is the right choice for me. The length of time in schooling, the cost of schooling, and the level of autonomy of a PA have only reinforced my decision. This is why becoming a PA is more appealing that any of the other provider roles.

I believe that my education and other life experiences have prepared me for a life as a PA. Working at a pediatric clinic has provided me with invaluable knowledge of the patient provider relationship. The clinic also provided me with a good foundation in symptom presentation, treatments, and diagnoses. Having physicians and nurse practitioners that were willing to explain diagnoses and treatments has enabled me to learn even more. Working at the clinic has also allowed me to improve my communication skills with patients. Communication is key to providing good care. My job consists of calling the patient back, recording their chief complaint, and then recording their vitals. All of this requires excellent communication between myself and the patient. I have to make sure I'm writing down the information the patient is giving me correctly. This allows the provider to get a preliminary idea of why the patient is being seen. My education, while tough at times, was very rewarding. My second year of college is where I struggled the most. I had just transferred and I hadn't fully realized the impact that my grades would make later on. I think this was an important learning lesson for me as I had to work even harder to get my GPA back on track. As the courses got increasingly difficult, I learned better study methods and was generally able to gradually increase my GPA. I managed to graduate with honors despite a few rough semesters.

With the new healthcare reform being put in place, more patients that ever will be seeing providers. It is important to me that the provider patient relationship remain intact. When there is trust between a patient and a provider, care is more accurate and meaningful. As a PA, it would be important to create a healthy and caring environment for patients because this is what keeps the relationship going. While I was shadowing one day, there was a patient who was following up after seeing her cardiologist. She insisted on hearing the results from the PA even though the cardiologist had already explained everything to her. She told me it was because she trusted her provider. To the patient, the PA was the only person who could adequately provide care for her because she was seeing the whole picture, not just one part of her body. After seeing how a PA functions on a daily basis, I know this is something that I want to do.

Commentary Essay 10

First, a couple of technical points — contractions are disfavored in academic essays, so I advise people not to use them except in dialog. You also make a common grammar error, using the singular (patient) and plural (their) of a noun in the same sentence. They're easy to miss, but details matter to Admissions folks, so double-check everything for grammar.

You have a solid essay — it covers key points, but could use livening up. To start, I'd skip the last line of the first paragraph. It is just stuck in without context and it sounds presumptuous. The third and fourth sentences of the second paragraph read like a job description. Eliminate those and add something like this, "I decided to shadow PAs to see if their role was as fascinating as the descriptions I had read." Then go into the information about Faith. But instead of just telling us about it, show us with a patient example. Show Faith dealing with the patient, interacting with the physicians, etc. That brings an otherwise dry description to life. The same applies to your clinic experiences. I know you can do this because you do it well in the conclusion.

I can't tell from this formatting if you have a separate paragraph about your education/GPA issues. But if it isn't one, it needs to be. You also need to transition to that paragraph, which by the way, could be shortened. A transition sentence might be something like,

"My clinical and shadowing experiences have been great preparation for becoming a PA. My education has been as well, although my early grades may not reflect this." Then go from there.

Essay 11

I was riding along in the back of an overcrowded van, seemingly lost in the prairies of western Ukraine. The pothole littered road made for a painfully unpleasant journey. Heat from the summer air caused beads of sweat to roll down each passenger's face. Most of these people had never been within 500 miles of an American, let alone sat next to one on a rutted ride to the village of Ostroh. As we traveled, I couldn't help but notice that nearly every passenger had an ailment of some kind. Two deaf passengers were animatedly speaking sign language to each other. An elderly woman had a dirty glass eye and an open wound on her face that desperately needed medical attention. Another passenger was sitting with crutches made from tree branches and a cleverly crafted cast wrapped around his leg using sticks and cardboard.

At age nineteen, I was asked to serve a two-year mission for The Church of Jesus Christ of Latter-day Saints. I was asked to serve in Ukraine; a country to which I had never previously given any serious thought. I did not anticipate that my journey in Eastern Europe would open my eyes to the needs of people living in isolated areas of the world. Riding along in that overcrowded van, my mind began to wander, thinking of how differently these people's lives would be if they had appropriate medical care available to them—especially with many of them still suffering health complications from the 1986 Chernobyl disaster.

It wouldn't be perfectly honest to say that this was the point in my life when I decided to be a Physician Assistant. In fact, I had no idea what a Physician Assistant was! However, upon returning home from Ukraine, I knew I had a passion for interacting with and helping people. My experience in that part of the world opened my eyes to what I wanted to do with the rest of my life. I knew that I needed to be in a field of study where I would give of myself to help others around me.

One year after returning home from Ukraine, my brother-in-law told me that he was considering pursuing a career as a Physician Assistant. As we talked, my interest was piqued, and I decided to look into it further. I had not previously considered a career in the medical field, and I felt as though a new door had been opened to me. I quickly found myself researching everything I could find about the profession and its history. It struck a chord deep inside of me. I frequently reflected on my experiences with the wonderful people in Ukraine who would have benefited from having Physician Assistants in rural areas. I had a newly kindled desire to reach out to people in medically underserved areas here in the United States, and to serve them to the best of my ability.

It was at this time that I changed my path in college. After enrolling in an EMT course, my eyes were opened to the world of medicine, and I fell in love with it. As I progressed through the EMT course, I wanted to expand my knowledge, skills, and scope of practice. The university I attended offered a program in Paramedicine, for which I applied and was accepted. Throughout the paramedic program, my vision of medicine was expanded, and my desires to help people through the practice of medicine were solidified.

I recall an experience I had on the ambulance late one night. We were called to an elderly woman who was having a significant gastrointestinal bleed. We quickly loaded her into the ambulance, administered fluids, and then had a lengthy ride to the hospital. During the ride, I had the opportunity to talk with this woman about her life. As we discussed her medical history, she shared how much she loved her Physician Assistant that she frequently visited at her local clinic. She spoke of his kindness, his generosity to take her calls after hours, and how he always took the time to educate and answer her questions. I was thrilled to hear that she had such a good relationship with her Physician Assistant and told her that I also had aspirations to enter the same profession. As we arrived at the hospital and said goodbye, the patient warmly smiled at me and said, "You are going to make an excellent PA." Those words have resonated within me and have given me motivation in times of difficulty.

From the time I spent in the villages of Ukraine, to the time I now spend as a paramedic, I've realized that my eyes have been opened for a reason. I believe that I am meant to be a Physician Assistant. I believe in making connections with patients. I believe in supporting, educating, and working collaboratively in this spectacular niche of medicine. I believe in making a difference.

Commentary Essay 11

Before I get to content, I'll point out a couple of housekeeping items. Contractions are disfavored in academic essays, so I advise people not to use them except in dialog. Don't capitalize physician assistant unless it's part of a formal name or a school specific essay that capitalizes it generally. You also need one space between sentences and you haven't always done that. It's minor, but fix it before you submit.

Overall, you have an excellent essay. I would avoid using the word "passion." It's so overused that it's virtually meaningless. And I think it's a bit dangerous to say you were meant to be a PA. Take ownership of your experiences and the decisions that brought you to this point. Unless you're applying only to schools that are religious based, I'd leave that type of writing out.

Essay 12

I am applying for the second time to become a PA I only applied to 1 school last year and I am on the waiting list at Texas Tech and wishing for a miracle to be accepted but if I do not I want to be ready and apply again here and to others schools. I do not know if I should resubmit the same essay or change some information any help I can get is helpful.

Fear, hunger, pain, death – these are all characteristics of the place where I was born: Huajuapan, a small town in Oaxaca, Mexico. An underserved community with few health resources to keep a premature baby diagnosed with bronchopulmonary dysplasia like myself alive, a place where socioeconomic realities impact medical access on those whose very life is on the line.

I was very ill throughout my childhood. The doctors recommended my mother reduce my exposure to potential infections. This was hard since there was an increase in cases of tuberculosis in my town. My mother, frightened of what could happen to me, did not want to take any chances. She left everything she had – being a nurse, friends, and family – to bring me to the United

States to receive better treatment. I remember the people I trusted to ensure my wellbeing as I was in and out of the hospital. They made an impression on me and from that time on, I knew I wanted to enter a profession in the medical field. I met many doctors and physician assistants during my care. Growing up in a rural part of town the PA seemed to spend more time with me than the doctor did, taking the time to know me on an individual level rather than just another patient. One night, when I was at the hospital, my mother had to work and I was alone. I started to panic; I had to be hooked to oxygen to relieve my anxiety. I remember my PA staying with me until I fell asleep. I have come to realize that I sincerely enjoy getting to know people personally and tailoring myself to meet their needs and that as a PA it would be the best fit for who I am and what I find joy in; helping others.

I met many people who endured a set of challenges that were not far unlike those faced by my family who came to the United States for better opportunities. Even though medical resources are available to everyone, many faced the fear of going to the hospital due to lack of money or language barrier. I encountered people who could have prevented a condition if it were treated at an early stage, but the fact that they did not have the funds to do so was their downfall. I remember seeing my mother use her nursing skills to treat neighbors who were sick. Even though she could not work as a nurse, an immigrant herself, she practiced to help others as she did with me when I was sick. The consciousness my mother passed on to me established my desire to serve individuals in need and humanity at large.

My hunger to succeed has been essential, shaping the person I am today. I have come upon many obstacles throughout my life;

nevertheless, I had a goal in sight to alleviate the pain and suffering of places like Huajuapan and other underserved areas. As a first generation college student, it was tough, but knowing that my family looked up to me for being the first one in my family to graduate with a Bachelor's degree motivated me even more to prove to them anything is possible. Committed to pursuing a career as a PA, I dedicated my time in the medical field.

Working directly with patients has made me more confident about becoming a PA. As an EMT, I love being able to help patients when they need it the most, but it bothers me not knowing what happens to them after they are out the ambulance and I wish to be involved in a more in-depth level. As a caregiver and interpreter for an elderly patient with Alzheimer's, I learned the importance of providing companionship, conversation and how much a language barrier could affect one when struggling to understand one's health problems. While volunteering, I came upon a conversation of a family who only spoke Spanish. The doctor told them to bring their daughter back immediately if her symptoms worsened, and otherwise to follow up with a doctor in three days. However, what her parents understood from the conversation was that they should wait three days to see the doctor. I quickly interrupted and interpreted to make it clear that they should return immediately if symptoms worsened. A week later the doctor came up to me and thanked me. It turned out that the daughter had appendicitis and came back the next day instead of coming in three days later when it could have been too late. As a medical interpreter, I am the voice of underserved communities, to gain full access to quality health care by understanding and communicating effectively.

To this day, the town where I was born still has very few resources; my grandmother passed away five years ago due to a lack of blood available for transfusion. The pain of knowing we shared the same blood type but being many miles away in order to arrive on time even to say one last goodbye is still very devastating. I became headstrong and determined. I realized that I want to help people, care for people, to practice in underserved communities, and give them a second chance; I was given one after all. School has taught me medical facts, but life has inspired me to become a great physician assistant.

Commentary Essay 12

First to answer your question. Anytime you reapply, you don't want to submit the same essay. For one, you need to update the information since you last applied so they know what you've done to improve as a candidate. Include work/academic/volunteer/even personal experiences to show your growth.

The opening sentence of your essay is very strong. The second sentence is incomplete, so right away there's a technical problem with your essay. Watch for those, because you not only don't want errors, you want to keep your readers moving along without stumbling.

The third paragraph is awkward and has some inconsistencies, such as when you say that medical resources are available to everyone, yet say people without funds aren't getting the treatment they need. If you're going to make statements like that, you'll need to tie in a solution that you as a PA can help resolve. Otherwise, it won't help your essay. Skip the lines about your mom in that paragraph altogether. They don't belong there.

On the positive side. You did a great job of tying your opening to the conclusion, and I love the last line. Wonderful job there.

Essay 13

As a child I was told that you should do what interests you, you should do what you love. Since I took my first steps my true love has been sports. To be honest, I can't recall what first drew me into the competitive arena. Perhaps it was because my parents were both competitive runners, or maybe there's some ancient DNA sequence within that programmed me to like chasing things. Growing up I played soccer and basketball, running intermittently in the background. I joined my school's crosscountry squad in sixth grade and running quickly became my primary sport. I am especially drawn to running because it showcases all of the things I love most about sports: competitiveness, mental challenge, and, in the case of track relays, collaboration with others. As my mileage increased each summer, so did my passion for running as a sport. After my sophomore year of high school, I stopped playing traveling basketball to focus solely on my endurance training. At the end of my junior year, my dedication earned me appointment as captain of both the girl's crosscountry and track teams at my high school.

Then, my senior year, tragedy struck. In the winter of 2010, I played on a recreational basketball for fun. During a playoff game I was knocked down and tore my ACL, swiftly ending my high school running career.

I didn't run a step for 5 months after the injury. I spent hours in physical therapy working to get back my strength so I could compete again. It was the most difficult period of my life to date. Thankfully I recovered very well from my surgery, though my journey back to running was a long process. I was able to compete my freshman year, though my training was very limited by my injury. I was patient, waiting until the summer before my sophomore year before slowly building up my mileage. Since then I have run personal bests in every event as well as set school records in several individual events and relays. These successes were well worth the wait.

Dealing with injury is a dark time for an athlete. Luckily I discovered a silver lining to my situation. Enduring a serious injury taught me to never take anything for granted, to always give my best and compete like it was my last chance. It also sparked my interest in Sports Medicine. My freshman year of college I arranged to shadow a friend of my mothers who works as an orthopedic physician. Dr. Voight entered each exam with a smile and gently led each patient through the tests necessary to diagnose their injury, gamely answering any questions and quelling any concerns they had. The day I spent following her on her rounds solidified my choice to pursue a career in sports medicine. Her positivity and dedication are qualities I hope to emulate in my future medical career.

After my day with Dr. Voight I wanted to begin building my experience in the medical field. Unfortunately, as a student athlete it was difficult to find a position that meshed well with my busy schedule. Luckily, I was able to secure a part-time position as a medical scribe in the Emergency Department (ED) and Urgent Care (UC) of a nearby hospital. I primarily work in Urgent Care, whose evening and weekend hours are a better fit for my busy schedule. This allows me to work closely with Physician Assistants. Working as a scribe the past year has not only improved my medical knowledge and vocabulary, but also made me realize that PA school is the right path for me. To complete another step towards my dream path I completed an Athletic Training class this spring. I look forward to gaining more hands on experience next year working as a Sports Medicine Assistant with the Athletic Training staff at Carleton.

As coaching great Bill Bowerman once said "running, one might say, is basically an absurd pastime upon which to be exhausting ourselves. But if you can find meaning in the type of running you need to do...chances are you'll be able to find meaning in that other absurd pastime – LIFE." My dedication to running led to one of the most difficult periods of my life, but it also improved my resolve and helped me realize what I wanted to do with my future. For the last ten years of my life academics and varsity athletics have been the center of my life. I look forward to moving on to the next phase and transferring my passion and dedication to a new area: my career as a PA in Sports Medicine

Commentary Essay 13

Before I forget, the technical items — contractions are disfavored in academic essays, so I advise people not to use them except in dialog. Don't capitalize physician assistant unless it's part of a formal name or a school specific essay that capitalizes it generally. Cross-country is spelled as I've written it, not as one word. Part time is two words, not one. Spell out numbers one through nine except when telling time and in ages.

Now for content. While this essay has some good writing, it has problems, starting from the beginning. When you start an essay for PA school by saying your true love and interest is sports, I'm wondering right away if you've sent in the application to the wrong place. Focusing almost exclusively on your running career doesn't allow you to cover what is really important in this essay, such as why you want to be a PA! I even think that calling tearing your ACL a tragedy is a mistake. Tragedies are death, devastation due to earthquakes, flooding, fires. Yes, it was sad and a disaster to your running career, but in this essay, you need to get out of yourself to focus on the call of the question — why you want to be a PA.

All you say essentially about that is that it's the right profession for you. Now you need to back it up with facts. Write what appeals to you about the profession and why. But don't do it as a job description, use examples. Instead of writing about your experiences with Dr. Voight in such detail, do the same with a PA. When I was reading the part about the doctor, my impression was that this was a med school application. Leave out the quote from the coach. We get that running is huge to you, but you have to convince your readers that you are sincere about becoming a PA.

Essay 14

I believe the people you encounter and the experiences you have shape who you will become. I believe I was born to be a healer, and throughout my life special relationships and experiences have led me to where I am today.

I was fifteen, lying on the cold floor of a hospital awaiting my friend to wake up from surgery after a terrible car wreck when I became absolutely positive I wanted to be on the other side of that situation. I was confident in that moment that I wanted to do everything in my power to make sure I would be the one helping others through the field of medicine. Unbeknownst to her, my friend's physician assistant that day helped me decide my life's future direction. I wanted to be her, a member of the medical team, someone who could alleviate the pain and heal the hurting; that's what I want to do for the rest of my life.

Throughout my undergraduate career, I was able to do just that after being given the opportunity to work alongside health professionals on a number of medical service trips. Of all trips, my most memorable trip was with Global Brigades to Ghana, Africa. The experience changed my life forever for the better. The knowledge I gained in medicine and the sweet smiles received from those who were helped in the clinics and even those who I simply encountered will be eternally imprinted onto my brain and my heart.

When we first arrived, my brigade team and I pulled up in a rickety old bus to an old dusty road and were greeted by dozens of welcoming faces from the community of Abor. As we stopped, the crowd ran over to us. Enthusiastically waving their arms as if they needed to get our attention. I hopped off the bus and immediately was grabbed by two small girls, one on each hand. I can still feel their small dirt creased fingers intermingled with mine. Honored, I looked down at them as they tried to conceal a smile and hide the great joy they had inside them.

Soon, our brigade group paired with translators and spread throughout the community going door to door to each residence to meet the members and hear their stories. The connections we made through the exchanges of smiles and laughter superseded what mere words could ever have conveyed. The language difference was not a barrier, but allowed actions and expressions to trump words, making the relationships between us stronger.

Two American doctors and two Ghanaian doctors coached us in identifying the cause of each patient's pain or problem based on not only their symptoms but also taking into account their living situations. After reassessing their vitals and symptoms, I asked the patient more questions to better understand what was going on. It took practice, but after a while I correctly identified the disorder and treated each patient with help from the brigade team and the doctors. I felt an overwhelming feeling of accomplishment and a rush of adrenaline run through me after each medical mystery (or so I liked to think) was solved. I thought of each symptom as a puzzle piece that fit into a big puzzle. The symptoms and living conditions (puzzle pieces) all correctly fit together to form the problem as a whole (the whole puzzle).

Some diagnoses were untreatable by our triage and those patients were referred to the hospital. I found myself frustrated when I could not do anything to help the patient, when the case was unable to be treated in triage. As a physician assistant I will do everything in my power to help in the treatment of every patient. As a physician assistant I hope to be there for my patients and to be involved with them through every step of the process until healed.

Leaving Africa was hard but I was comforted that the efforts of Global Brigades would continue and that my time working in healthcare was only just beginning. My trip to Africa opened up my eyes to what medicine can do. The people of Africa reinforced my desire to always demonstrate commitment to community and dedication to family. The optimism and cheerfulness found within even the sickest of the sick in Abor was moving. I want to carry on their tradition of community, dedication and joy through service to others in medicine. I want to become a physician assistant not only to help alleviate the pain in others but also to inspire as those in Africa inspired me.

As a physician assistant, I would be able to help those in need of health care. The unbearable pain faced by many could be treated with my help. As a Physician Assistant, I could help change the world and stop the suffering; that is my prime motivation. As for now, I plan to continue my medical work as a certified nursing assistant, serving others while living and traveling throughout Australia. I look forward to the time that I can gain more knowledge and training as a physician assistant to help those all over the world in need of medical care.

Commentary Essay 14

First, start your essay with the second paragraph. It is engaging and compelling and I was immediately hooked. The first paragraph is what I call throat clearing — you're getting ready to write what is really important. In that second paragraph, now your first, change this: I wanted to be on the other side of that situation" to this "I wanted to be on the health provider side of that situation." Otherwise it's confusing. Then you can eliminate the next sentence (it's redundant) without losing the message.

Watch for those generic type sentences. This is another: "The knowledge I gained in medicine and the sweet smiles received from those who were helped in the clinics and even those who I simply encountered will be eternally imprinted onto my brain and my heart." You're wasting valuable characters/spaces on something that doesn't say much of anything. And it actually sounds sophomoric to say words like "will be eternally imprinted onto my brain and my heart." Things similar are: "Honored, I looked down at them as they tried to conceal a smile and hide the great joy they had inside them." That sentence doesn't say anything about your experience. And how do you know they were trying to hide the great joy they had inside, or if they felt joy for that matter. I'm not trying to be mean about it, but you really want to make every word count. For that reason, you'll leave out the paragraph that starts with "Soon our group brigade..." (You wouldn't want to start two paragraphs with "Soon," anyway).

Now that you have the room, you'll write about what's really important in the essay that's missing— why you want to be a PA. I thought you were going to tell me about your friend's PA and what she did to convince you that was the career for you. That's what you need to do with that PA or others. Yes, the essay says you want to be a PA and includes some things you could do as a PA, but you're lacking the specific details about why you want this career in particular. If you didn't have enough contact with your friend's PA to write details, then use other experiences — shadowing, any volunteer work that involved PAs, other personal experiences or work experiences with PAs if you have it. That will make all the difference for you in this essay from being a generic sounding piece to a compelling one.

Essay 15

I ran down the steps with two baby pictures in my hand. One of these pictures resembled me, the other did not. I was only seven at the time so I asked my mother who the other baby was. It was then that she said three simple words that would change my life. "You were adopted".

Hurt and confused I ran and hid away from my adoptive parents because in that split second they had become strangers. The other baby girl was their second adoption option at the orphanage. I should have felt lucky at that moment, but the revelation created a void full of feelings of isolation and uncertainty that caused me to question who I was.

Luckily, I grew up in a close knit community and this helped to mend my feelings of isolation; however I still felt something was missing. I knew where I belonged, but did not know my purpose. My community was not only close knit but also encouraged giving back by donating volunteer time and money to implement change and help build friendships. It was through the volunteer work and my job at a local bank, that I was able to rebuild my sense of identity and claim my purpose. I was blessed with a second chance at a better life and I want to now share that with the world. I want to be a physician assistant so I can give back to, and build healthier communities with acts of kindness.

My desire to give back to my community was vital in guiding me towards my volunteer, education and job choices. In my youth I volunteered for human rights associations like CAIR (The Council on American Islamic Relations) and Salaam Cleveland. CAIR has been essential in bridging connections between people of different faiths in our community and defending the rights of those who were violated. At an event held by Salaam Cleveland, I was able to help sick children by preparing meals at Ronald McDonald House Charities while they received medical treatment at the Cleveland Clinic. I also volunteered at Health Fairs for the underserved and refugee communities of Cleveland. The fairs gave me a glimpse into the affects poverty can have on a person's health. At these fairs I helped by promoting the events, and registering the participants. These experiences further validated my desire to help my community. Influenced by my volunteer choices, I chose to pursue a degree in political science. Both my education and my job choice were influenced by my volunteering experiences. I worked at a bank as a teller which helped me pay for my education. The job was not glamorous, but it taught me how to foster relationships with my customers and improve on my soft skills. At this point I was considering law school and I continued to work hard to get good grades. After graduating magna cum laude, I realized that I desired a more personal interaction with people and was not partial to spending copious amounts of time immersed in paperwork which lawyers often do. Promoting community, diversity, and justice are not limited to the political arena; they also play a major role in med-icine.

On this expedition towards becoming a physician assistant, my shadowing experiences have been the final decision maker. I no-ticed that doctors hardly spend any time getting to know the patient and in some cases do not see the patient at all. With all the advances in healthcare, I know that positive human interac-tion makes the biggest impact. One of the most touching events I witnessed during my shadowing experience was that of a five year old girl's Jtube reinsertion. As she held tightly to her fa-ther's hands, her tears and small cries affected all of us in the emergency room. I was in awe of the compassion shown to her by the physician assistant who aided the doctor. In that moment, I realized that this is my calling.

I used to shy away from telling people that I was adopted, how-ever that act of kindness done by my parents was one of the best examples of giving back to the community. They opened their hearts and home to someone who they owed no dues. One day when they are old and frail, I hope to be able to repay them for everything they have done for me. Taking care of my parents has taught me essential life lessons that will be beneficial when it comes time to take care of my patients. Becoming a physician assistant would provide me with the opportunity to create healthy communities by building relationships with my patients and providing them with individualized care all while maintain-ing their autonomy. It would also reiterate my own sense of purpose. I am no longer that hurt little girl with feelings of iso-lation and uncertainty. No longer does doubt plague my thoughts. I had to find myself before I could define myself and it was through my educational, volunteering and job experiences that I attained certainty. I know I possess the qualities required to be a successful physician assistant, not only academically, but also humanistically.

Commentary Essay 15

Grammar, grammar, grammar — quotation marks always go outside the end punctuation. It's not, "You were adopted". It's "You were adopted." You'd write five-year old instead of five year old. Although you're not paying me to be picky today, that's the specific kind of advice I give when I edit. Grammar is important — When I interviewed Admissions Directors and faculty across the country about writing these essays for our book, "How To Write Your Physician Assistant Personal Statement," all said there shouldn't be any grammar errors, that it was a red flag that people didn't pay attention to details. In healthcare, missing the details can lead to death!

Now onto the content.

Your essay is quite well written from a technical standpoint, an advantage you have right off the bat. And the opening is quite engaging. But after reading the first couple of paragraphs, I had the feeling you were estranged from your parents, and the only way you felt less isolated was engaging in the community. I suggest you approach it from a positive perspective instead of the negative. While as a reader I was happy to see you volunteering and connecting with your community, I felt really bad about your parents, and that detracted from everything else. I probably won't be the only person bothered by this. You can still tie in how your community helped you feel connected, but include your parents in this positive experience somehow. I'm sure they were part of it. We shouldn't have to wait until the end to see that you are still connected to your parents.

Finally, we don't know how you got from political science to medicine. What led you to consider medicine? It's a big leap from the case law studies of law school to the blood and guts of PA school regardless of the way you try to explain it here. You'll need to be specific so we understand your journey. And although human interaction is key to the PA's role, it is not unique to that profession.

You could be a CNA, an MA, a nurse, an NP or even a social worker for that matter. You'll need specific reasons to explain why you decided to be a PA that go beyond patient relationships. Use your patient example, but expand on it.

Essay 16

The streets were filled with garbage and the stench from it was overwhelming. Children were roaming the streets by themselves, while traffic on the roads was creating their own sort of noise. I began to wonder why we even came here in the first place.

It was in the summer of 2003; through young, innocent eyes, those were just some of the images that were front and center as we drove from the airport through the poverty stricken area of Hyderabad, India. Although I was only eleven at the time, witnessing extreme poverty for the first time was a surreal moment. To make matters more interesting, it was also the place of my birth.

Several homes were clustered together; others were more like shacks held intact with cardboard and plywood. As my family drove further along with the intended destination being my aunt's house, my bewilderment grew upon each street we entered. Prior to arriving in India, I had known only a life filled with relative ease; this was in stark contrast to the lives of the children in Hyderabad, many of whom lived in those clustered houses. Several of these children had no parents, little food to eat; yet it was awe inspiring to see them smile through all of their transgressions. During the course of our twomonth stay in Hyderabad, my aunt would often host these underprivileged children at her house; she would provide them food and clothing from donations she collected within the neighborhood. Without hesitation, my aunt had allowed me to assist her with the children. It was during this time where I learned the true meaning of giving what little you have to others. My family continued to return to Hyderabad several times throughout my childhood. With each visit, I was increasingly perplexed and troubled as to how such disparities in lifestyles can exist and at the same time, I was continuously inspired by the compassion shown by my aunt in continuing to serve the disenfranchised. It was through these experiences early in my life that planted my desire to spend my life serving others.

By the time I had reached college, I wanted to pursue a profession that was catered around helping others. It was not until when I got my first job as a pharmacy technician that I began to develop an interest in the field of medicine and health development. It was also at this time that I enrolled in Rollins College majoring in International Relations and International Business. Obtaining a liberal arts degree allowed me to become a better-rounded individual capable of trying to address the most pressing issues we face in the world today, particularly that of international health development. In order to translate my desires into an actual profession where I could pursue my dreams, I began to conduct research on careers in health care that would fit this exact criterion. Soon enough, I came across the description of the role of a physician assistant and I was immediately drawn to it. It would allow me to interact with patients one on one and get to know their story, which is something I highly value. It would require academically challenging science and health related coursework, which I enjoy. Even when out in the workforce, it seemed a physician assistant would never stop learning and had ample flexibility in the settings they could work. All of this was appealing, but what truly drew me to the career was how essential physician assistants are in offering primary care to underserved and rural populations. I was instantly reminded me of my aunt, who selflessly serves everyone in her community, and now I can have the opportunity to one day to the same. Growing up in a tightknit community, I have seen a strong need for accessible primary care. I had a family friend who passed away from a cancer that could have been caught with routine screening, a friend with severe type II diabetes that was diagnosed after months of neglected symptoms, and the list goes on and on. Having seen the negative outcomes of health care disparities, I am excited and honored to one day serve my community by working to provide accessible health care.

Immediately after deciding to pursue a career as a physician assistant, I began to shadow a Physician Assistant and a Medical Doctor at a local urgent care clinic. At the clinic, I was able to perform urinalysis, electrocardiogram, physical exams, take vital signs, and even write prescriptions all under the supervision of the PA and the MD. The knowledge that I have gained through the handson experience at the clinic was priceless, as I was able to interact with patients from all backgrounds. Working at the clinic was done in simultaneous fashion with working at the pharmacy; this allowed me to become current with the latest drugs in the pharmaceutical industry. With these experiences and several other shadowing and clinical experiences, my choice to pursue a career as a physician assistant has only been confirmed.

I have chosen to become a physician assistant because I feel its role and purpose resonates with who I am and what I value. I desire to help people lead healthy, productive lives and have seen how crucial the role of primary care plays in that. I have seen such a need for accessible health care in my rural community and desire to help in meeting that need. This is the need I am passionate about; this is where my service makes me feel alive.

Commentary Essay 16

Before I comment on the content, I need to point out that your essay is more than 300 characters/spaces over the CASPA limit. You need to make sure you've cut to under the maximum before you submit or your essay will be cut off wherever the limit hits. Again on the technical side, a couple of words are joined together — at least how this came through in the formatting. So if you know better, I apologize for the following corrections: Betterrounded is two words (better rounded) as is handson (hands on). Twomonth is also two words, two month. Finally, you wouldn't capitalize either Physician Assistant or Medical Doctor.

Luckily, it won't be hard to get under the CASPA limit because there's a lot of passive writing. To make the first paragraph as striking as it was in real life, you could write something like this instead: "The stench from garbage-filled streets overwhelmed. Children roamed alone, ignoring the smell and noise of the cars cramming the roads. I wondered why we came here in the first place."

In the second paragraph, you could eliminate the year because you gave your age. You only need one or the other. And you could significantly cut that paragraph. We don't need the detailed descriptions — save the space to use for the more current events — the shadowing I talk about below.

Resist the temptation to give a laundry list description of the role of the PA—use your shadowing experience to highlight the things that appeal to you and are important. The exception is the part about physicians bridging the gap so to speak in healthcare in underserved areas. That ties in with the theme of your essay.

Essay 17

As the daughter of an operating room (OR) nurse and certified nurse practitioner (CRNP), I am fortunate to have my mother as such a strong role model. She showed me how hard work and serving others results in a rewarding career. She works on weekends and takes call in the OR in addition to her full time job as CRNP. On the other hand, I am the daughter of my father, a paranoid schizophrenic. In first grade, I can recall asking him repeatedly to take his medication, but he always refused, due side effects from the medication. I remember him telling me over and over about satellites in the sky and the dangers of the radio and the church. I spent a majority of my life trying to understand my father's condition to explain his behavior to my friends. Not having a "normal" dad was hard to accept. At the time I was not aware, but looking back this experience first drew me towards medicine. I was constantly observing, evaluating, and explaining my father's disease.

Only after college did I really understand the biological cause of my father's disease. I wanted him to take medication, as I continued to witness his auditory hallucinations. However, he denies any affliction of disease. I've learned to accept him, listen to him with patience and respect, and spend quality with him. He spends a lot of time in the garden, plotting plants and herbs into particular geometric shapes into the entirety of the back yard. He is happy and content. I've learned that my fathers' best interest is the most important, not mine. I've also learned that not only the patient's life is affected, but also the family members. I now try to remind myself to empathize with and treat each patient I interact with as if that person were my mother, father, or any other family member.

I continued my involvement in medicine with a 2year fellowship at the National Institutes of Health (NIH) in Nursing Research. Here, I was exposed to many different health professions nurses, doctors, researchers, rehabilitation, and physicians' assistants. Attending the prostate multidisciplinary clinic weekly at NIH really led me towards the physician assistant (PA) career. Each patient was discussed among a team of doctors and the PA to determine the best plan of treatment based diagnostic tests. I was intrigued by the complexities of each case, and how the "best" plan could easily change, depending on disease progression and the patient's decision. New research affecting treatments revealed to me that medicine is not an exact science and requires a lifetime of learning. From here, I succeeded in acing the remaining PA prerequisites on top of my full time job. I became a certified nursing/geriatric assistant and joined Georgetown Orthopedics as a medical assistant (MA).

As a MA, I have found fulfillment in my work, as well as a natural propensity for fixing and finding solutions to mechanical complications, regarding to splinting and casting. I have also found that I am very limited. After listening to patient's frustrations, problems, and fears, I would like to also diagnose and treat patients. I take every opportunity I have to ask the doctors about certain treatments. For example, why immobilization is better then surgery, or how a certain injury would have implications down the road, and why certain medications are prescribed. I want the knowledge to read images and review reports to correlate clinically. The PA in our office also serves as the first assist in surgery, which I would love to get my hands on. PAs are devoted to their patients, which motivates me to become one of them. The need for PAs in our society is increasing and our population is continuing to get older. Working with patients has given me the desire, willingness, and determination to further my education in order to provide the best and appropriate care.

Thank you for your consideration and allowing me the opportunity to follow my dream

Commentary Essay 17

I was sorry to read about your dad. I know the heartbreak and frustration that comes with the disease. But it does give you a great opening, which you do very, very well with a couple exceptions — leave out the acronyms in parentheses and omit this sentence: "She works on weekends and takes call in the OR in addition to her full time job as CRNP." You don't need it and it takes away from the impact of what comes next. Also, in this sentence: "In first grade, I can recall asking him repeatedly to take his medication, but he always refused, due side effects from the medication," you left out the word "to" after "due" in this sentence, and you could leave out "from the medication," because it's redundant. You don't want grammar errors — they matter greatly to Admissions folks as they told me when I interviewed them, and especially in the first paragraph! There are a couple of others, including using "then" instead of "than."

You could eliminate most of the second paragraph. We don't really need the details about your dad's daily life or that you kept trying to get him to take his meds. What we need from that paragraph is the insight that you write about so well. So leave out the sentences after the first one until the one that starts, "I've learned . . ." (only don't use contractions — they're disfavored in academic essays and skip the parentheses for the acronyms for PA and MA while you're at it. Anyone reading these essays knows what they stand for).

And leave out the last sentence of the essay. It detracts from the strength of your conclusion.

Other than those points, the essay is very well done. You do a great job of saying why you want to be a PA and outlining your experiences that will contribute to your success as one.

Essay 18

It's 2:30 in the morning and I am finishing up my shift, when a man runs into the lobby yelling for help, "My friend is in the car and he can't move!" I hurry outside and find a man in his thirties looking at me with a helpless stare. Without hesitation, I grab security and we lift him into a wheelchair. I alert the nurse and have a code stroke paged overhead. Working together, we get the patients blood work, EKG, IV and CAT scan done within fifteen minutes. The CAT scan shows an ischemic stroke that will need a clotbusting medication to treat. After a tense two hours the man miraculously regains sensation and speech. As I recheck his vital signs, he is slowly able to grasp my hand, and through a thick Spanish accent, whispers, "thank you". It was this moment that I realized I wanted to work in healthcare for the rest of my life. The feeling of achievement was better than any victory I have ever felt. I am striving to become a physician assistant because it would not only give me the conduit to make a substantial difference in peoples lives but it would provide me with an ultimate sense of fulfillment and purpose.

Long before I knew what a physician assistant was, I was rambunctious six year old, kicking around a muddy soccer ball in the backyard. I would beg my younger sister to play goalie while I sent shot after shot spiraling toward her face. Although soccer isn't the focus of my life anymore, it is the foundation of my character. Through it, I gained strong teamwork and leadership skills, as well as a scholarship to the University of San Francisco. It was here where I cultivated a fervent fascination towards medicine through my exercise and sports science major.

After a successful academic career, I returned home eager get a certificate as an Emergency Medical Technician (EMT) so I could gain valuable healthcare experience. In my time as an EMT working in an Emergency Room, I have seen patients go into cardiac arrest, assisted a ventriculostomy and even helped deliver a baby. Besides these remarkable clinical exposures, I have also been able to interact with numerous doctors, nurses, and PAs. These conversations confirmed my decision to apply to physician assistant school.

After researching the differences between midlevel providers, I decided that I wanted to practice under a medical model instead of a nursing philosophy. However, I still needed reassurance that becoming PA would be more fulfilling than being a doctor. I remember the positive response I got when I told one of the female physician assistant's I work with that I was thinking about applying to PA school. She compared her career satisfaction to a doctor she knows that has had to sacrifice substantial time with her family in order to stay competitive in her career. I find the healthy work life balance of a PA much more appealing. I am also interested in the ability to change specialties throughout my career. I believe having an overall sense of life fulfillment will allow me to care for my patients at a deeper level.

A major source of my gratification is found via interactions I've had with those who suffer from disabilities. Growing up alongside a close family friend who has downs syndrome influenced my desire to build relationships with others like her. One of the most memorable activities I did in high school was mentoring a young girl with autism. I have continued to find other opportunities like this throughout college and beyond. Last summer, I volunteered at a summer camp for children with spina bifida and cerebral palsy. I was moved by the positive outlook these children displayed toward life despite being confined to a wheelchair. My aspiration to practice medicine, where people desperately need quality healthcare, developed from the involvement I have had working with these inspiring individuals.

Last application cycle I applied to a few programs however, reflecting on that decision I understand I was not ready to be accepted. I applied late, had courses in progress and I barely surpassed the healthcare requirements. These technicalities aside, I realized I was not confident enough to take on the challenges expected of a PA. Another year of preparation has increased my medical knowledge and improved my poise around patients and providers. Taking more science courses has also readied me for the academic rigors of PA school.

My extensive background in athletics has qualified me for a career that is teamwork oriented and allows me to pursue other meaningful endeavors. I know my strong clinical experience has shaped my knowledge of the physician assistant profession as well as my maturity to handle this responsibility. Moments of gratitude I have received from patients during their life-threatening emergencies, have unleashed my deep desire to dedicate my life to providing quality healthcare.

Commentary Essay 18

Good job on the opening — it's engaging, action packed and has the perfect amount of drama. If it weren't for the grammar mistakes — "patients" instead of "patient's," end quotation marks inside the punctuation instead of outside and "peoples" instead of "people's," I wouldn't change a thing. There are other mistakes throughout the essay, and don't use contractions in academic writing.

I can't emphasize grammar issues enough. Although I know this is a draft, catch them as you write so you won't miss them later. They really do matter to Admissions folks, who expect these to essays to be free of grammar mistakes.

In that second paragraph, you need a bit broader scope. So instead of this: I was rambunctious six-year old . . ." do something like this: "I was rambunctious kid kicking around a muddy soccer ball in the backyard, a high schooler who gave every free minute of her time to the game and a collegiate competitor." Skip the sentence about your sister. It's cute, but doesn't add anything.

The rest of the essay is very well done with an exception I'll get to in a few lines — you explain what you've done in the year since you last applied. Admissions folks definitely want that information, you tell about your experiences and humanize them and tell why you want to be a PA. Here's the exception — I really don't think it's wise to say you want to be a PA because of life balance. If you were on an Admissions Committee and had two equally qualified candidates, would you pick the one that said, "My career is my everything to me," or the one who suggested she prefers the 8-5 type of job? It's an exaggeration of course, but think about it.

Essay 19

As our plane touches down and grinds to a halt the cabin erupts into enthusiastic applause. Being a frequent flyer I wonder what the fuss is all about. A friend leans forward from the aisle behind me and says; "Now I'll tell you. This airport is considered one of the most dangerous in the world because the runway is so short. After a deadly accident in 2008, it was lengthened a few hundred feet and the limited pilots flying here have to undergo specialized training." At this revelation I was ready to join in on the praise for our pilots and safe landing.

We had arrived for a weeklong medical mission trip to treat the humble people of San Antonio de Flores, a small, mountain town in Honduras. It was my first trip and my thoughts were filled with wonder and anticipation. From our mission home base it would be a four hour bus ride, traveling up and down tortuous dirt roads to where we would set up our clinic. I would serve as part of the triage team, measuring weights and taking blood pressures as we checked in patients. Fortunately—and for security reasons—triage was stationed near the only door. This gave us the opportunity to be the first faces of welcome and to also say goodbye to the thankful patients carrying bags full of much needed medications, shoes, eyeglasses, etc. It was incredibly rewarding to witness firsthand the impact we were having.

I have been contemplating my career choice as a physician assistant for many years now. As a teenager, our neighborhood clinic was mainly staffed with PAs so our family has long been comfortable turning to them for our healthcare. Relishing the hard sciences, I have always desired a career in medicine. I was able to determine early on however, that I did not want to be a medical doctor. Despite the tempting salary, I felt the lifestyle was not a good match for me. With my husband joining the military and plans to start a family, the typical workweek and student debt of an MD were demands I did not want to force myself to meet.

More recently, I have taken a position as a patient care techni- cian at The Nebraska Medical Center to broaden my understanding of the allied health professions. Understanding that nurses play a vital role in the wellbeing of a patient, I still feel compelled to learn medicine based on the medical physician model. Thinking back to the first day of clinic in Honduras, one nurse commented, "It's as if we're functioning as doctors and PAs, even though we're nurses; it's a little overwhelming." I un- derstood her apprehensions and as the days passed, the nurses did become more relaxed. These concerns however, only further cemented my belief that I have chosen my true calling of service.

In opposition to my current maturity, my behavior as I started college was admittedly quite the display of irresponsibility. The actions I took in my freshman and sophomore years were defi- nitely those of a selfish adolescent. I was not focused on my schoolwork and my disregard for the dormitory rules led to a one year disciplinary dismissal from Texas A&M University. Ini- tially, I was determined to return, but after attending my local community college and gaining steady employment in a restau- rant—where I met my husband—I decided to complete my undergraduate degree at the University of North Texas. With great family support, galvanized focus, and a deeper respect for my studies I graduated Cum Laude with a Bachelor of Science in Biology.

Today, as a proud military wife and mother of two I am ready to advance my career and learn how to provide excellent healthcare. The collaborative relationship between the PAs and MDs greatly motivates me. So much can be accomplished with continuous feedback and open communication. As a primary healthcare provider, I want to dialogue and teach preventive medicine as well as help diagnose and treat illness. The broad spectrum of specialties open to a graduating PA holds great value for gaining experience and skills. I am faithfully eager for knowledge and want to pass along that knowledge to meaningfully help the underserved.

Commentary Essay 19

This is a really excellent essay. You've covered the bases and done it well. That includes the dismissal from Texas A&M. The one thing I caution about it is to say you wouldn't want to be an MD because you wanted to start a family and didn't like the typical MD's work week. That makes it sound as if you couldn't be a mom and a student or a doctor, something that could put off or even offend members of an Admissions Committee. If you were on an Admissions Committee and had two equally qualified candidates, would you pick the one that said, "My career is my everything to me," or the one who suggested she prefers the 8-5 type of job? It's an exaggeration of course, but think about it. Certainly there are other differences you could write about — the ability to spend more time with patients, the opportunity to provide patient education, etc.

Which reminds me of one more thing — don't ever use "etc." in an essay like this. It's lazy writing. These essays are all about specific details.

Essay 20

In his book Wishful Thinking: A Theological ABC, Frederick Buechner exhorts his readers to search for "the place where your deep gladness and the world's deep hunger meet." He says that this is the place to which we are called, our vocation. I have found my vocational calling in the multifaceted role of the Physician Assistant.

As a relational person, I thrive on meeting new people, conversing with them, sharing in their life stories, and encouraging them to seek wellbeing. I enjoy getting to know others on a deeper level, seeking growth and meaningful relationships with those I meet. I had the pleasure of pursuing strong and lasting relationships as a Resident Assistant at Calvin College. During this experience I was the leader and role model for younger students and learned many lessons in how to interact and encourage others. Similar to Resident Assistants, PAs are given the opportunity to enter into deep relationships with people—experiencing their hurts, fears, and addictions, but also their joys, healing, and families. My favorite experiences while shadowing PAs was watching them interact with patients. Each PA I observed treated their patients with the highest care and respect. They actively listened to the patients' concerns, thoughtfully answered questions, and anticipated patients' needs. It was clear that these PAs loved people and worked in a profession that allowed them to give physical and emotional care to their patients. As a PA I would cherish the opportunity to enter into my patients' lives and work hard to understand them, recognize their values, and strive with them toward healthy living.

However, being a high quality PA goes far beyond a listening ear and caring heart. It requires medical knowledge and the ability to aid patients in understanding their own medical conditions. My fascination with the intricate mechanisms of the human body stimulates me to study diligently and to seek a deeper understanding of how the body works. In short, studying the body, its structure and functions, excites me. In turn, this knowledge allows me to educate my patients, explaining to them how their bodies function and how various treatments and lifestyle choices will affect their specific conditions. Through my experiences at hospitals and health clinics, I have seen that when patients have a clear understanding of their own situations they feel empowered to make informed decisions and are more likely to take ownership of their health. My interest in medicine and my skill in teaching at each person's level of understanding further reinforces my desire to take up the PA's role, a profession which leans heavily on patient education and empowerment.

Medical education and high quality care are particularly important to vulnerable patients, which often includes those living in medically underserved areas. People living without adequate access to medical providers, those living in poverty, immigrants, and patients who suffer from longterm disabilities may experience unnecessary illness due to irregular care, lack of financial resources for treatments, or inadequate understanding of preventable conditions. A PA's extensive medical knowledge combined with clinical experience and relational skills makes the PA's role well suited to serve these populations. As an added benefit, PAs can lean on the extensive knowledge of the team of medical professionals with whom they work, promising better overall care for their patients. My experiences living abroad, working with urban, impoverished patients and the chronically disabled, as well as my undergraduate studies in development have both fueled and led to my desire to work more closely with underserved populations. I care deeply for these populations of people and fully desire to see them reach places of joy and satisfaction in their lives. I believe that the PA profession will best allow me to serve the underserved, and I am deeply committed to providing excellent health care and expertise.

My desire for longterm relationships, enjoyment of medicine and patient education, and commitment to the vulnerable and underserved leads me to pursue the PA profession. I am convinced that I will excel in this profession due to my personal character, professional experience, and willingness to apply myself diligently to the tasks of continual learning and patient care. I truly believe that the PA profession is where my "deep gladness and the world's deep hunger meet".

Commentary Essay 20

Well, if you're going to quote, you'd better do it right! You didn't give the whole quote, and the way you wrote it suggests that it is. Either add the rest of the words or use ellipses to show it's not the whole quote. Apart from a few other technical issues, which I'll get to in a moment, the content and flow of the essay are great. You transition between paragraphs and even sentences (your readers will value that), and you clearly write why you want to be a PA and why you'll be a good one. So excellent job there.

Here are my picky, but important points. The use of the word, "relational" is one. Even if you could use it as an adjective, it will stop your readers and make them wonder what you're talking about. You misspelled the word "stories," make long term one word when it's two, and in the last sentence, put the end quotation marks before the punctuation, which is a grammar error. Another grammar error, although common, it to use the singular of a noun (a PA/a patient) and the plural (their) in the same sentence. Grammar/spelling errors matter to Admissions folks, because as they told me, missed details can mean death in healthcare. Fix the things I've mentioned and you'll have an essay to compete with the best of them.

Essay 21

I am passionate about my pursuit in becoming a physician assistant because there is little room for compassion towards suffering patients in the American health system and other health care systems around the world. There is something unfortunately ironic about a profession that's basic purpose is to help others and yet many times, that is the opposite of what takes place within healthcare and medicine. When I become a physician assistant, my highest priorities will be to show compassion and to increase my patient's role in their own healthcare by helping them understand their health conditions. The goal of the PA profession's origin, to improve and expand healthcare, is a cause I am zealous about promoting. This is why I am pursuing a career as a physician assistant.

One of my earliest exposures to the downfalls of the American healthcare system was in middle school. I remember riding to the hospital with my grandmother for her medical appointment. When we arrived, the office staff was overwhelmed by the amount of ailing and scared patients. They were too overrun to answer questions or provide comfort to anyone checking in. Once we were brought back to a patient room, I made a trip to the restroom while we waited. Upon exiting the room, I heard the medical professional mention my grandmother's name and saying "why is she here again?" followed by "I don't have time to comfort people." I vividly remember that floral wallpapered room with my grandmother sitting on the paper covered table and all I wanted to do was help her escape from the unsympathetic person that saw her as someone filling an appointment slot.

However, on my high school mission trip to the beautiful island of Cuba, my eyes were opened to the medical conditions in other countries less fortunate than ours. During the trip, our group met a woman named Elena who shared her story with us. She had previously been diagnosed with ovarian tumors. The medical team working on her case had tried a few available treatments but none of them seemed to improve her condition. Finally, the head medical professional on the team determined that a hysterectomy was the only viable solution to her problem. Elena described wearing her favorite worn, blue dress on the way to her procedure and was surrounded by several friends and family who were there to provide support. After hugs and kisses, her support system waved as Elena was wheeled off to the operating room. Elena explained that she had heard anesthesia had been in low supply around the hospital for a while but no medical professional on her team had actually mentioned this to her. However, she was successfully put under anesthesia to begin her surgery. As the surgery proceeded, she began to wake up and feel excruciating pain. She says that she began trying to motion to let someone know she was waking up and says that she was told by someone in the room that the anesthesiologist was gone and she remained awake for the rest of the surgery. Although that only was a couple of minutes, she said that felt like a lifetime. Elena told us that although that was several years ago, she vividly remembers what it felt like to not be shown any compassion while lying on the operating table. She ended her story emotionally by saying, "I thought I was supposed to trust them to care for me." Elena and her story have stuck with me throughout the last few years as I have worked professionally, academically, and socially towards my pursuit of becoming a physician assistant.

While some key characteristics to being a physician assistant include intellect, observation, and communication, I would place a greater emphasis on exhibiting compassion, integrity, and concern for my patients. I want to increase the understanding that patients have about what is actually going on in their own bodies, instead of just handing them a prescription without explaining how it will affect them and their health. How can we gain a patient's trust if we do not take measures to earn it? This is why I am passionate about becoming part of this profession that can make all the difference in a person's healthcare experience.

Commentary Essay 21

You make a point that has truth to it — some healthcare providers lack compassion. And certainly it can be said that healthcare systems are not designed with compassion as their primary goal. However, your essay's opening is so negative, it's truly off-putting. I'd delete the opening sentences you get to this, "The goal of the PA profession's origin, to improve and expand healthcare, is a cause I am zealous about promoting. This is why I am pursuing a career as a physician assistant." That turns the negative into a positive and clearly states a proactive goal."

I'd skip the part about your grandmother altogether. Really, there are many kind, compassionate healthcare providers, and focusing on the negative doesn't help your essay. There are two reasons — one is that you'll come across as a negative person who sees only the bad things. Equally important, a need for compassion isn't unique to the PA profession. You could be a compassionate NP, MD, MA, even a social worker. As to the Cuban trip, instead of making it a damning example of insensitivity, use the example to talk about the lack of resources and training and how you'd work to combat that as a PA.

When you write this:" While some key characteristics to being a physician assistant include intellect, observation, and communication, I would place a greater emphasis on exhibiting compassion, integrity, and concern for my patients," I worry that Admissions folks will think you're disregarding key components of the profession. The things you say are less important deserve equal weight to compassion, integrity and concern. You'd be a poor PA without those things!

After reading the essay, I don't know why you want to be a PA as opposed to another career. What specifically attracts you to the profession? How will it allow you to reach your goals of improving and expanding healthcare that other careers won't? Those are the questions Admissions folks want you to answer.

Essay 22

I have been raised from a young age to seek out knowledge. One of the first things I attained was a thirst for facts about the human body. My love for cars brings out this analogy for the human body. I describe it as akin to a car with the heart being the engine, the oil being the blood, and the gasoline as the nutrients. All of these components (with many more added) are essential to the survival and function of the machine/organism. From a functional standpoint, both the car and human body are incredibly complex and share a similar design. They both use energy to perform work. When a component fails in either the human body or a car, it can be difficult to diagnose and repair the problem. There is a deep seated fascination within me to understand and diagnose any problems that might occur with the human body. I have studied many different books and have taken several classes underlying the anatomy and physiology of the human body. All the learning I have done over the course of my childhood delves into the didactic aspects of medicine.

When I was a junior in high school, I took the PLAN test that was a part of the ACT. The results of that test were that I would be best suited to working with people. In order to find out if a career in medicine is right for me, I searched for a position that would allow me to delve into the clinical aspect of medicine. Recently, I started volunteering as a Spanish medical interpreter at Community Health clinic. My primary job is to allow for the both the patient and doctor to communicate with each other. I am voice of the patient to the doctor. I am the patient's advocate and their conduit for receiving medical care. Working alongside the medical professionals, have helped me realize that medicine is my true calling. The experience of working in this clinic has assured me that the underserved and underprivileged can receive medical care and should receive medical care. The clinic provides me with the opportunity to give back to the community, and also to learn the skills and demeanor of a medical professional. It is truly the best of both worlds volunteering at this clinic. I am blessed to be associated with such an organization.

As a first generation college student, there was always the yearning to become a doctor. I was going to be the first in my family to not only graduate from college, but also earn a medical degree. This was before I even knew about the career choice to become a Physician's Assistant. A career as a Physician's Assistant will allow me to work autonomously, but yet have a guiding hand in moments of need. I want a career that will stimulate me and allow me to have a family while also having time to see to their needs. A career as a PA strikes a balance of time and commitment that I desire out of a career in medicine. This career also allows me to continue to explore and diagnose the anatomy and physiology of the human body. It will give me the ability to freely choose a specialty and move around different specialties in order to enhance my knowledge in the field of medicine. I am also hopeful, that being a PA will give me a chance to serve my community and underserved populations. A Physician's Assistant program will prepare me for a rewarding and lifelong career track.

Commentary Essay 22

You make a fatal error in your essay, and that's getting the name of the profession wrong. It is never, ever "physician's assistant." It is physician assistant (not capitalized). So before you do another thing, correct that everywhere. If you have it wrong here, it's probably wrong in your application and resume, too.

Congratulations on being the first in your family to graduate college and to pursue a medical degree. It's huge for you and your family. But in order to be the first in your family to be a PA, your essay needs to get you an interview, and the way it is now won't cut it.

First is the car analogy. You could use it if you carried it throughout the essay, but there's no other mention of it after the opening. You'd need a clever tie-in, something more than your love of cars. I'd probably start the essay with your second paragraph, which is a disarming introduction to you.

When you talk about wanting to be a PA, I'd definitely leave out the part about lifestyle benefits. I really don't think it's wise to say you want to be a PA because of life balance. If you were on an Admissions Committee and had two equally qualified candidates, would you pick the one that said, "My career is my everything to me," or the one who suggested he/she prefers the 8-5 type of job? It's an exaggeration of course, but think about it.

Also, it really sounds as if you just read about PAs online. Instead of listing things about the profession that sound like a job description, bring it to life. Have you worked with or shadowed PAs, or had one as a provider? If so, use those experiences to describe what you saw that appealed to you about the profession. Describe how the PA interacted with the patient, the supervising physician, other staff, family members. Say why you want to do those things and why you'll be good at them. That will show you know what the profession is all about and why it's right for you.

Essay 23

Remember that wherever your heart is, there you will find your treasure."

— Paulo Coelho, the Alchemist

I have learned over the years that difficulties we face in our lives shape our personalities and make us grow. I would not be the person I am now if I did not learn to overcome obstacles of my past. When I got sick and the doctors could not determine exactly what the diagnosis was I felt devastated. I thought I did not deserve it and there should be a way to resolve it. When I finally found a doctor that gave me hope, I was truly delighted and hopeful. She had a plan of treatment and it was the beginning of a new life for me. Once I got cured, I had a strong desire to help people to be healthy. I realized that I wanted to be that one person that could give hope and make a difference in the life of others.

Over the years I worked in various medical clinics as an acupuncturist and a nutritionist. I educated patients on prevention of the health problems and on proper diet plans. When one of the clinics needed an extra medical assistant, I was willing to get a proper training to help. That job was an eye opener since I had to participate in the life of patients who were in a need of a complex care. I realized that I wanted to be able to make a bigger

contribution in their life. I started researching different opportunities in a medical field. One of the doctors suggested looking
into a PA program. After doing a research on a history and responsibilities of the profession I was inspired to follow this path.
I shadowed Medical Doctors, Nurse Practitioners, and Physician
Assistants to understand a world of medical providers and their
differences.

I feel that everything happens for a reason if we make our experiences become our best teachers. Last year my newborn baby
spent three weeks in NICU and it was the most exhausting and
fearful time of my life. I had a chance to see PAs and MDs providing an exceptional care, knowledge, and research on my child's
condition. We had a great PA, who took the time to educate us,
to listen to our concerns, and to make an extra step to provide us
with options and information regarding child's health. I feel like
being a parent and going through the struggle for my child's life
tought me patience, gave me extra strength and maturity, and
made me feel closer to people who are in the same situation.

Shadowing Janai, PA in pediatric orthopedic surgery department, inspired me to keep following my dreams. She showed me
what a great PA should be. I was impressed by her knowledge,
devotion, and willingness to help and work in cooperation with
other team members. Being a mother, I felt heartbroken for children that had serious congenital health problems or complex
aquired conditions. I thought that treating complicated health
problems on a daily basis would make you a thick skinned and
less compassionate. I was really surprised when Janai told me
that she never lost that feeling. She told me that kindheartedness
actually makes you a better health provider. Her words strengthened my desire to become a PA and confirmed that it will be the

best fit for me. I admire her attitude and her great contribution to the life of others.

I know that becoming a PA is a challenging and demanding road. I do believe that I have the qualities to be an honorable student. My determination and tenacity keep me focused on my goals and finish the projects I start. Last year I managed to take my final in genetics three days after I had my child. My teacher was impressed and told me that I showed a great example of commitment to other students.

I want to be a PA that encourages and inspires others and I am grateful to PAs that were my mentors without knowing it. I place confidence that my devotion, compassion to others, hunger for knowledge, and, most importantly, sincere care for others will make me an extraordinary Physician Assistant.

Commentary Essay 23

This is a very compelling essay, and well-written, too. You show great heart, but with great restraint. The essay could have been sappy or over-emotional and it's not at all. Great job!

That's not to say it's perfect. You've capitalized Medical Doctors, Nurse Practitioners, and Physician Assistants when they shouldn't be, you write "life" where it should be "lives" more than once, and have spelling errors — "tought" instead of "taught" and "aquired" instead of "acquired." Admissions folks don't look kindly on these errors as minor as they seem — missed details or errors in a healthcare situation can cause disaster.

Other than fixing those issues, I wouldn't change a thing. Great work!

Essay 24

In biology class in 2011, my teacher, Dr. Misayah, provided an answer to a lifelong quest I have had for wellness and healing compassionately, and effectively.   She described how she was delivering a pregnant woman at home who did not have health insurance and didn't want to go to the hospital. The woman was not expelling the placenta. Dr. Misayah used her fingers and gently separated the placenta to avoid hemorrhage from tearing the uterus. She saved the patient's life.   I saw in that moment how my mother, who died when I was 30, could have lived. She was a German immigrant who had survived the war and spoke only broken English. She was someone who simply needed extra compassion and caring before she could trust, and seek help. She had a stroke, refused to go to the hospital and died at home. I have gained an increasing perspective on that tragic loss for myself and my family as I have grown older and pursued differ- ent paths, and I now know that my passion is to work with medically underprivileged communities who need that extra kindness and understanding to help recover from illness and lead healthy lives. I had heard of the Physician Assistant (PA) profession from a friend, the role of the PA, and of the work that would be entailed, and now saw how it could all fit together. Dr. Misayah's story galvanized me to become a PA.

Since that moment of realization, I have been preparing for this profession with a focus and drive that exemplifies who I am. From a young age, I have thrived on challenges. When my dad retired from the Air Force and we settled in New Mexico, I de- cided at the age of 12 that I wanted to be a gymnast. We didn't have money for me to go to college, and although I knew I was starting late, (most people who are successful at gymnastics start by age 6), I applied myself with a tenaciousness that allowed me to get a full scholarship at age 17. I maintained that scholarship for five years of my undergraduate studies. While in college, I was exposed to music, which led to my becoming a professional singer/songwriter. I applied the same principle of determination, and as happened in gymnastics, I was successful. I became the lead singer for a nationally recognized band, toured extensively, and am currently awaiting the release of my 8th CD. I have connected to people through my music specifically for the purpose of mental and emotional healing, and that satisfied a very deep need I had, but there was still something important missing. While I have explored other areas to apply myself as an adult, including teaching, becoming an accomplished practitioner and yoga teacher, and a talented chef, I now know that I want to be involved with people at a more critical level, contributing to their health and wellness. The height of service for me is being the kind of healthcare practitioner my mother would have come to for help. I want to care for people by being part of a healthcare team devoted to helping save lives and improve the health of those people who are reluctant to ask for help for reasons such as poverty or immigration status.

I have taken my preliminary studies seriously, with the same approach to challenge as before, and although I am far from finished, I have begun to apply the many acquired skills and abilities that I have. One of the most rewarding experiences I have had so far came from using previous knowledge of movement and anatomy from my yoga training. I detected a slight abnormality in the gait of one of my current home health care clients that indicated a potentially serious problem. I was able to see that although it wasn't a stroke or blood sugar issue, it required more than rest, and necessitated a visit to the hospital. It was discovered he had a blood clot in his leg, and my concern and attention to detail averted what could have been a tragedy.

Through my nontraditional background, I bring a wealth of knowledge in a number of fields, and a personal and professional maturity, to the work of being a PA. My previous life experiences as a gymnast and musician have taught me the value of communication and teamwork. The same concern for the health, wellbeing, and compassion for others, that has informed all I have done, will inform my work as a PA. I believe this variety of experience forms the basis from which I can make a distinctive contribution to the PA healthcare field.

My long-term goals as a PA are twofold. First, I hope to work in medically underprivileged communities, contributing on teams of medical professionals who are also moved by compassion and empathic understanding of others' life situations to serve their patients. And second, I aspire to use what I learn as a PA to help educate future generations of PAs. I have the commitment and motivation necessary to succeed, as well as the desire and compassion that drives me to want to make a difference in the lives of others.

Commentary Essay 24

I was very sorry to read about your mom. Sadly, for immigrants who are untrusting or unfamiliar with healthcare here, it is not an uncommon occurrence. On the positive side, congratulations on your CDs — it's no small accomplishment to produce music.

Your essay has some good writing, but the opening paragraph has too much going on — there's Dr. Misayah, your mother and that you decided to be a PA. For one, I didn't see the connection between this: In biology class in 2011, my teacher, Dr. Misayah provided an answer to a lifelong quest I have had for wellness and healing compassionately, and effectively," and the rest of the paragraph. The answer is not tied in, even with the sentence, " She saved a life." And it really has no tie to why you want to be a PA other than she saved a life. That's not enough to carry the statement. So the example doesn't do the work you'd hoped.

If your theme is that you hope to work in medically underserved communities, I'd stick with your mother's story for the entire opening paragraph. It's very compelling. That would require additional rewriting to transition to the next paragraph.

I'd also resist the temptation to add the laundry list of other careers you've tried out. Music and gymnastics are fine, but when you go on, I begin to wonder if becoming a PA isn't just another career to try and discard. If I wondered, others will, too. Save those other things for when you're asked about outside interests.

Finally, you need to say more about why you want to be a PA. You talk quite a bit about why you'd be a good one, but not why you want to be one in the first place. Expand on that from what you've observed PAs do on the job, if possible. That will help bring the reasons to life.

Essay 25

Strip a person of all worldly belongings. What remains is the body and mind. These are the things manipulated by healthcare providers. It is an incredibly intimate honor to be so trusted with that responsibility. Some providers take this for granted while some patients offer their trust thoughtlessly. I do not claim to understand it completely but I remain cognizant that what I do affects people, sometimes in a very profound way. I take this lesson with me in all aspects of my life because integrity is one of my most coveted virtues. My motivation to become a physician assistant (PA) blossoms from embracing this trust and responsibility to ameliorate suffering and vivify the lives of the patients I encounter.

Working with animals in the animal hospital was the first time I became interested in healthcare. The hours I spent every week leaning over the shoulder of the veterinarians and technicians inspired me to enroll in an emergency medical technician (EMT) class. I practiced as EMT throughout my years studying illustration. As time and experience changed my priorities, I began considering health care as a career instead of a job.

Although illustration is a far cry from medicine, art has taught me the balance between the details and the whole composition. Just as you cannot create a successful painting concentrating on one subject, you cannot heal the whole body without considering all its systems. Spending three hours a day critiquing student work has taught me the value of criticism, the wisdom of experience, and the innovation of outside perspective. Most pragmatically it gave me a solid foundation of anatomy. Being in an open studio community taught me to learn from and teach my peers which I continue to do today as a CPR and lab instructor for EMT students. Teaching to me is almost the equivalent of learning because it demands mastery of the material and managing people. Each class is different and as always in medicine, the science and technology changes daily.

My greatest influence has been my work in the city as an EMT. Mostly, EMTs treat symptoms but one of our greatest skills is our assessments to find underlying pathology. Sometimes finding the pathology is readily evident but more times than not, the pathology becomes challenging to diagnose and treat for many reasons. Information collected can only be gained on scene, from bystanders, and from the patient. Diagnostic equipment is limited. Treatments are exclusively impermanent, albeit life saving interventions. Working within these constraints has refined my resourcefulness and ability to think and react under pressure. As a PA I could amend many of these restrictions by being a part of a team, with collective knowledge and experience, without completely sacrificing autonomy.

One of the things that is thoroughly taught in EMS is patient advocacy for their social, mental, and medical health. As an EMT this means working with the family, bystanders, fire department, police, and health care providers to effectively treat and transfer a patient to definitive care. Even if that only means notifying the correct authorities and passing along information. Above all it means conferring understanding to the patient about their health, educating them, and giving them tools to improve their own life as well. As a PA I can do infinitely more through healing, education, and advocacy than I ever could as a nurse or paramedic.

On scene, the middle age woman was slurring her words, combative with the police, and ataxic, though notably lacking the smell of alcohol. "I was just drinking water, they wouldn't let me watch the game!," she said after exiting the bar with a police escort. It was not until I took her medical history that I discerned the real problem, hypoglycemia. The police assumed she was lying. We talked about where she lived and how often she monitored her diabetes. Because she had been staying with various friends, her glucometer and strips were lost. She hadn't checked it in a couple weeks. I gave her oral glucose en route to the hospital and quickly expressed my concern to a nurse once we arrived at the hospital. The nurse seemed distracted at first but my persistence was rewarded. Her blood glucose was 20 g/dL. It was busy that night. Patients were doubled up in rooms while beds and chairs lined the halls. What if she had been put in a chair and left alone to fall asleep? Before leaving, I notified social services and walked by her bed which now featured empty cups of orange juice. When her eyes found me she thanked me, words muffled by a turkey sandwich.

When I see how trusted PAs are with patients and physicians it strengthens my resolve to pursue this career. Either working or shadowing I have seen how PAs have made the difference in someone's life in not just a diagnosis and treatment but in compassion and understanding. A multitude of experiences have prepared me for this path. I want to be profoundly part of people's lives.

Commentary Essay 25

Your essay has much to commend it, but not the first paragraph. It's very confusing. The problem is not uncommon even among experienced writers. We have a thought and think we have written it clearly, only to find that the clarity is in our minds and not on the page. We are not grounded in the facts in your opening paragraph. For example, I have no idea at that point what you do that affects people or how you affect them.

When you say that healthcare providers manipulate body and mind, my initial impression is that it's a bad thing. Manipulation has a negative connotation. And I don't see how integrity is connected to any of it.

This sentence: "Some providers take this for granted while some patients offer their trust thoughtlessly," doesn't make sense to me at all. I probably won't be the only one struggling with it.

Start with the second paragraph. It's got great information and is well written. It tells us in a couple of sentences how you got into healthcare, why and is a great lead-in to all the benefits you've gained from your art.

You also need a transition to your paragraph with the patient example (a good one to choose on many levels).

But other than those complaints, I have none. The essay covers all the key issues for these essays and does it well.

Essay 26

A heartbeat is what bring moments of our life to come together, my fascination of a heartbeat did much more than that. During my elementary school years my father had a suffered heart attack, he required a triple bypass operation. The unfamiliarity and skepticism led me to seek more knowledge about the heart. Which led me to creating this heart model, made from plastic tubes, pumps and paint in my school science fair in elementary school.

After acquiring my phlebotomy certification I had decided to go volunteer at North Shore Long Island Jewish Hospital. I decided to walk in to the volunteer department and sign up but had forgotten that I had my scrubs on after coming from my EKG class. As I was leaving the hospital grounds I bumped into a man, he had this smile of relief on his face as soon as he saw me. He then came up to me and said "Thank You So Much Doctor my wife is recovering so much better after the splenectomy". My confused faced turned around in hopes to see a surgeon standing behind me, instead there was no one but myself. After a while the man had realized that he had mistaken me as a Surgeon. For that very brief moment of his realization I felt this overwhelmed feeling of appreciation even for something that I didn't do. That sense of accomplishment and saving a life had given me that understanding as to what a surgeon must feel after performing surgery in an operating room for hours. This patient's husband had made me reassure myself that I needed to continue on my path towards becoming a physician.

I had decided on becoming a doctor in my undergraduate years. After completion of my Bachelors I decided to take up a position as a phlebotomist/laboratory technician to further my clinical skills. At Bellevue hospital my job was not only to interact with the patients in drawing blood but also being able to see the specimen sample afterwards as it would undergo the necessary tests needed. This allowed me to observe the doctors as well as to what tests were ordered and when doctors would monitor patients with certain illnesses. My interaction with the patients allowed me to practice my bedside manner and I had the opportunity to meet with some of the Physician Assistants. I was able to observe how they interacted with a patient and became more intrigued by the role of a Physician Assistant as I had seen in the case with my father, the physician assistants' were the one to spend the majority of the time with the patient as well as decide on the treatment and discharge the patients at the North Shore Long Island Jewish Hospital. I saw how the physicians held the physician assistants' decisions in high respect and rarely change the orders.

The constant thought in my mind raised the question, what truly is the limit of a Physician assistant as opposed to a nurse practitioner or a physician. My respect grew more for when I was shadowing a Physician Assistant. This experience has clarified my image of a physician assistants' role in health care, as well as given me a better understanding of where I hope to be in this field. A physician assistant is able to adapt to a different specialty with less restrictions as opposed to a physician whom requires years of practice within that specialty.

The rhythmic patterns of a heartbeat show the very challenges of life with its ups and downs. Facing various challenges when it came to my father's condition and supporting my family in their time of need. I have grown through my clinical experiences and have chosen the correct path that proves to be challenging and rewarding at the same time. I know that becoming a PA is a demanding road and I plan on overcoming those obstacles I will face.

Commentary Essay 26

I was sorry to read about your dad's heart attack. How frightening as a child. It's a powerful subject to start an essay with, but here, you didn't do it the right way. The opening paragraph simply doesn't work. Here are the problems:

- The first sentence doesn't make sense (in addition to being grammatically incorrect — it should be two sentences).

- What does your fascination with a heartbeat have to do with either the first sentence or the rest of the paragraph?

- What were you skeptical about, and why would you be skeptical about anything you'd written about so far?

- How does creating a heart model in elementary school connect to why you want to be a PA. (That sentence, in addition to the other problems was incomplete).

So start with your dad's heart attack if you want — often it is a traumatic childhood experience that starts someone on the path to healthcare provider. You can even start the essay with the sentence about heartbeats you have in the conclusion, modified as follows: "The rhythmic patterns of a heartbeat mirror the very challenges of life with its ups and downs." Tell about your dad's heart attack next and why it made you interested in the human body and medicine. Then go from there.

The next problem is literally what comes next. There's no transition to the second paragraph. You know how and why you decided to be a phlebotomist, but we don't. Tell us.

I like the example you gave about the patient's husband mistaking you for a surgeon. It's humorous, and I understand how it made you want to continue pursuit of a healthcare career. But you've got to get the grammar correct. The quote should read like this (and note where I have the end quotation mark, which is where it should be): Thank you so such, Doctor. My wife is recovering so much better after the splenectomy."

The essay starts to pick up when talk about your job at Bellevue and how and why you decided to be a PA. There are a couple of small problems here — don't capitalize physician assistant and only use apostrophes when you're using the possessive of the word. There are other grammar errors. Beware of those.

If you use the heartbeat sentence in the opening, you can keep still keep it in your conclusion. I like the repetition because it's a compelling sentence. In the conclusion you'd add something about overcoming the challenges of life's ups and downs. By the way, the second sentence in the conclusion needs to be fixed. It's an incomplete sentence.

Essay 27

I used to run. Not jog or sprint, but run. For 50 miles or more, I would run on streets, logging roads, and mountain trails. I rarely felt more peace and freedom than on a trail, sweat dripping and muscles fatigued, watching the sunrise. I found that there were few places in the world where a person could learn more about themselves than alone, pushing their body, surrounded by nature. Then, rather suddenly, running was no longer an option. One strong pull on a length of fire hose, and I was reduced to tears, forced to be held up by my crew because I could not walk on my own. My once strong body that I had pushed so often, that had taken me to the most beautiful places that nature had to offer, had betrayed me. Unfortunate genetics and years of punishment in the fire service had dealt me three herniated discs and a drastic change in my life plan.

My orthopedic surgeon told me that I can still be healthy, but a long career in the fire service would be out of the question. As I reflected on my future, I considered an experience I had a couple of years ago on an EMS call. We were treating a mother with an eye tumor in her small apartment. She needed to be transported to the hospital for treatment, but she was too ill to take her two small children with her. As a crew, we decided to stay with the children until their grandfather could come to the home. After helping the mother to the ambulance, we surveyed the apartment. It was small and sparsely furnished, but well kept. The mother had vomited on the carpet several times and we knew no one would be there to clean up for at least an hour, so we went to work. We scoured the house for cleaning supplies and toys to entertain the children. While we cleaned up, we played trains and hide and seek with the kids. Eventually, the grandfather arrived and thanked us for our help. After ten years in the fire service, I was reminded that day of why I had started a career in public service, to serve the public.

I have had many professional ups and downs during my short career, at times leaving me feeling jaded, overworked, and abused by the public. At other times, I have felt like a hero who was given the key to the city. My time running trails helped me develop positive characteristics, the greatest being perseverance. I cannot continue to work as a firefighter/paramedic, but I will continue to serve. I may not be able run those same trails, but I will continue to hike them. I will do my best to be a positive influence in my patients' lives every day. That is how I will continue to run.

Commentary Essay 27

The essay has many good things, but not enough. The words "physician assistant" don't even appear once. That's a problem in an essay that is supposed to say why you want to be a PA. You have some work to do to make this essay complete. You have to write why you've chosen the PA profession — you can write well, and have given a good patient example, so do the same using a PA. With that example, point out the things that resonate. What appeals to you about the role of the PA? Why not stay an EMT? What can you offer as a PA that you can't as an EMT and why does that matter to you? When you've added those things, you'll have answered the call of the question.

Essay 28

Room 345 is the room that changed me forever. It was just like any other day, and I had already ventured in there multiple times throughout my shift. During each visit, I took the time to talk with her, the patient, and her husband and got to know about their life — about their children, their marriage, their friendship, and their love for each other. We laughed and shared jokes, and I bid them farewell, until next time. I felt unbelievably at ease with them and I appreciated their kindness and the simple relationship we quickly formed.

At around 9:30 p.m. it was time for her last troponin to be drawn and was close to the end of my shift. I remember walking to her room, thankful that I knew what I would be walking in to — a pleasant, happy person who didn't mind that I was coming in there to perform what others find extremely uncomfortable and invasive: drawing her blood.

I walked into the room and headed over to the far bed. Something didn't feel right, didn't look right. She was uncomfortable and having difficulty breathing. I wanted to do something for her, whatever I could. In the blink of an eye, with her husband standing next to me, she was gone. I called for help immediately. As doctors and nurses ran into the room, I walked her husband into the hallway. A code blue was called overhead, which meant more people would soon be running into the room, causing her husband's panic and fear to run wild. I tried to relax and assure him that the staff was doing all that they could. She was not the first person I had watched take their last and final breath, but it was the first time I had watched a person take their last breath with their lifelong partner standing next to me. This pained me.

It was then, in that hallway that a rush of anger and desire took over me. I felt angry because I knew that there was nothing that I could've done, other than what I had done, at that moment of her distress. I am not trained nor qualified to run a code or assist in a code to revive a patient; nor am I trained to do anything more for the woman who I had grown fond of. However, it was also in that moment that a feeling of desire took over my anger, a desire to step out of the hallway and into the shoes of someone trained to handle and assist in situations such as these.

As her husband and I stood outside Room 345, a man, with whom I was familiar, came running down the long, cream -colored hallway toward us. It was Dr. Frazier, one of the head oncologists at McLaren Macomb. I remembered the woman told me earlier that day that she was having trouble with her heart and a blood clot. Seeing Dr. Frazier, I then realized she also had cancer.

I have always been heavily interested in both cardiology and oncology, but when I look back at my years in the health care field, I know this was the day and moment that solidified my desire to not only become a Physician assistant but to excel and train vigorously in one of these specialties. I do not dismiss what I provided for her husband that evening. I believe my presence, as someone to stand next to instead of standing alone was my purpose at that moment. The memory of this evening, every time I walk into room 345, and every other patient who has touched my life over the past 7 years is what motivates me to be exactly who I aspire to be.

Commentary Essay 28

I was engaged from the beginning with this story. It's excellent, but it's not enough. I have no idea why you want to be a physician assistant, which by the way should not be capitalized. Yes, you want to train in cardiology and oncology, but you could do that as an MD or nurse. You need to specifically tell why you are picking the PA profession above others. From reading this as it is, neither I nor anyone from an Admissions Committee know.

Essay 29

Acute Lymphatic Leukemia, and a look of terror on my mother's face. Out of everything the doctor said, and all the events that transpired when I was in the hospital that day, that phrase and my mother's face are all that I vividly remember. That's when I knew that something was really wrong. Sure, before that I knew that I was sicker than my older brother had ever been, but at 6 that still doesn't seem too bad. I soon found out how bad it actually was.

After three major surgeries, probably thousands of pills, seemingly endless blood work, and almost ten years I know how bad it was. I know that I am lucky to be here. Throughout my sickness there were many events that molded me into the person I am today and helped me decide that I want to pursue a career as a Physician's Assistant (PA). I had amazing Doctors and nurses that oversaw my treatment and I can attribute much of my desire to pursue this invaluable field to these amazing men and women. Ironically, one of the most significant and influential events in my recovery was orchestrated by a nameless face in the crowd of health care providers that oversaw my recovery.

At the tender age of seven I found myself sitting half naked on an operators table waiting for the surgeon to implant a PortACath next to my heart. As I sat there in my terrified and vulnerable state, a lady came up to me with an unknown object in her hand. "Are you ready for today's flight captain?" I had no idea what she meant. "I have your flight mask right here and whenever you're ready we can get the preflight checkup underway." She then proceeded to tell me that we were going on a beautiful flight over the mountains and that I just needed to put on my mask and we would take off. I relented and allowed her to put the "captain's flight mask" on me. She then sat behind me in the copilot's seat and we took off. As we soared with outstretched arms she described the beauty of the scenery we passed and I transformed from a frightened little boy to a confident pilot conducting my aircraft across a beautiful vista. Shortly after our flight lifted off the anesthesia flowing through cotton candy scented mask took effect and I faded into the horizon. I never knew that lady's title or even her name, but her actions as a copilot that day have molded me into what I am today. My decision to pursue a career in healthcare wasn't immediate, but when I did decide that I wanted to work in the medical field, she helped me understand why. I want to bring hope to the downtrodden and help heal the sick and afflicted.

As I grew older and matured, I came to realize the significance of the events that transpired through my youth and decided to pursue a career in healthcare. The problem I came to was simple: what area of healthcare would best suit me and enable me to achieve my desires to bring hope and healing to those in need. The possibilities were nearly endless, and I didn't really reach a decision until halfway through my undergraduate career. I was tutoring a well respected cardiologist's son in chemistry and calculus. Various circumstances made it to where the only place we could work was in the break room of the cardiologist's private practice, which happened to be right next door to the cardiologist's office. This particular tutoring job was invaluable because it enabled me to observe how a physician and a PA interact on a daily basis. As we delved into subjects such as Le Chatelier's

Principle and integrals I was able to listen to how patients were dealt with and which healthcare provider gave which service. I was astounded to discover that the majority of patient healthcare provider contact was through the Physician's Assistant. After gleaning this information I decided to research what a PA was, and the more I learned, the more I knew that if I wanted to fulfill my goals of bringing hope and health to those in need, then becoming a Physician's Assistant was the best path for me.

I will be a great Physician's Assistant because I will do for my patients what the unnamed lady did for me in my time of weakness. I will take them in their most vulnerable and scared state and help them become confident and ready to fly their own plane through their ailments. I will be able to do this because I will be able to have true compassion for them. Compassion is one thing that a book cannot teach. It only comes from being able to relate to others situation. I can help my patients because I know what it is like to have little hope. I know what it's like to spend weeks in the hospital. I know what it's like to suffer from severe sickness. I also know what it's like to overcome against all odds and to turn from an innocent frightened kid on an operating table to a confident, healthy person. My compassion will enable me to relate to my patients and bring hope to the downtrodden, and the wealth of knowledge I gain through your Physician's Assistant program will enable me to heal the sick and afflicted.

This is my rough draft, so I know there are some typos and probably some grammatical errors that need to be polished. Any input on content and flow would be much appreciated!

Commentary Essay 29

You have had an amazing experience, and you're smart to open your essay with it. However, neither that or anything else you have done will matter one bit if you don't get the name of the profession right. It is physician assistant (not capitalized and doctor isn't either), not physician's assistant, ever, under any circumstance!

As to the rest of the content, although your personal story is compelling, you don't want it to take up the bulk of your essay. The essay really needs more specifics about why you want to be a PA. At risk of sounding skeptical, I wonder how you were teaching Le Chatelier's Principle and integrals, yet during these sessions were not only hearing confidential patient/provider conversations, but observing the physician/PA interactions as well. It just doesn't ring true. So you'll need to do a better job of explaining all of that, especially if that's your only experience with PAs. If you've shadowed or worked with PAs, write about those experiences. You're a good writer and know how to bring a scene to life. Do that with a PA and his/her patient to exemplify the reasons you're choosing the profession.

One more thing — this phrase and the earlier variation are trite: "and bring hope to the downtrodden, and the wealth of knowledge I gain through your Physician's Assistant program will enable me to heal the sick and afflicted." I know you are more creative than that!

Essay 30

I was 10 years old and hospitalized for a peritonitis for about 3 weeks. Terrified and alone, I was begging for someone to explain what is about to happen to me, to clarify what is the doctor saying, and mainly to understand my fear.. and that's when a PA walked in and changed my life forever... Julie provided me a sense of calm and genuine comfort, she gave me a doll and showed me on the doll what the surgery was all about, I cherished it till today for that doll is what gave me my initial taste for medicine intertwined with a passion for human relationships. I was mesmerized by the wonder of the human body. At that age I had already and literally devoured a kids biology book and learnt it by heart. Science had always been my strongest point in high school and college. "Book smart", they would say. No, my good grades were fueled by a deep passionate love for understanding my surroundings, nature's elements, human body and human behavior. In Canada, schools provide the students with this program called HOPS, where students are invited in hospitals and shadow doctors, surgeons, nurses, etc. My high school did not offer this amazing program so I insisted on instilling it in my school for I was determined to attend it. Turned out that there was no more room for my school to join that year but I made everything possible to at least being able to attend the conferences. Being able to learn about each types of doctors and nurses, it only fueled me with this indisputable goal in life, that I want to be part of this big medical family that makes people's life better while allowing me to learn more about the human body which encompasses everything from math and physics to physiology, anatomy and chemistry . In high school I was enrolled in after schools program such as "friendship circle" and "Chai lifeline" where I dealt with sick and handicapped kids while helping their families, in the hospitals and in their house. This was another life changing experience which has brought me to really admire the role of PA after my countless encounter with them. "Aurelie, you would make a great PA one day!", my supervisor told me after helping the family of little 5 years old Ethan another innocent victim of cancer.

My early summer jobs consisted of working in the CDL laboratories. Again, simply to understand and being in touch with the complexity of my surroundings. In the lab, I learnt a lot about medicine first hand as I have never before, although the lack of human contact taught me that it should be a crucial part of life. This ability of excelling in human relationship building has brought me to open my own summer camp at the mere age of 16 years old, every summer until today. It took a lot of determination and organization to make this camp the success that it is in my community and especially to gain the parents trust of giving me, a 16 years old, the responsibility of their precious child. From organizing outings, bus, staff meetings, rent and all day dealing with kids has taught me a whole spectrum of valuable lesson in my life. Determined, passionate, creative, diligent and a very good team worker I know that Iv'e got what it takes to fulfill my dream of becoming a PA. Although, I am not afraid of rejection. Iv'e encountered many obstacles in my personal life which have a carved me into an even stronger person and all my challenges taught me not to be afraid of anything. I know in my heart and soul that that is what I am meant to do and I will do everything in my life to make it happen. I am a person that wants this title for the sole purpose of being able to bettering people's life while being able to study the subjects that I am simply in love with. I am choosing a PA over a NP after many hours of contemplating and researching both, but I have come to the conclusion that a PA have a greater ability with its more expanded license in disease prevention and developing a long term care plan with its patient. Not too long ago, I accompanied my father through the night to our local hospital ER. We were submitted at 9 o'clock at night and only have been seen by a doctor at 8 o'clock in the morning without any PA, nurse or anyone to give my dad a painkiller that he so terribly needed. The ER was surpassed and 1 doctor only treated 32 patients that night and 3 of them died.

That only exemplifies the need for PAs. Today, I am married and my loved one experienced great medical issues for a period of 3 years with ulcer colitis. As I have listened to his stories and experiences with hospitals and caregivers, how his PA literally have not only saved his life but also saved his morality and dignity, it only continues to fuel my already existing fire to belong to this precious group of angels better known as Physician Assistant.

Commentary Essay 30

You have great passion and heart, which are important traits in any health care provider. Those things come through in your essay.

It's missing quite a bit, though, particularly about your current experiences (apart from those with your family) in the healthcare field. Schools will definitely want to know if you've worked in any aspect of healthcare or volunteered in a clinic, for example. If you haven't any adult experiences, I suggest you try to obtain some by volunteering.

Even without those experiences, there are ways to focus your essay that will help convince Admissions folks to consider you. Based upon my interviews with Admissions Directors from schools across the country, I can tell you they aren't really too interested in much info about your childhood and high school experiences. Skip the childhood bout with peritonitis and spend only a couple of sentences about your high school experiences. Schools really want to know what you've been doing recently.

Starting and continuing to run a summer camp is impressive. It shows you have leadership skills. What else have you done in recent years? What about your college work? Did you focus on the sciences? Did you have internships? Spend time at hospitals?

There are some grammar errors, too. Do a spell and grammar check on your essay, and have others read it to make sure there aren't errors.

Essay 31

When I looked down all I could see were dark clouds sweeping up the valley like a tsunami of cold and rain; bad news for two rock climbers a thousand feet off the ground in the Canadian Rockies. Decision time. Do we risk the weather and try to finish the last 500 feet to the summit or do we pack it in and rappel down 5 hours' work climbing up Ha Ling Peak with little chance of attempting the climb again? We argued for too long and soon realized we were now subject to the whims of the fickle spring weather in the Rockies. We headed down in the cold and the wet, wishing we had left sooner. While in the uncomfortable embrace of disappointment and a climbing harness, I had no idea that this moment would set the foundation on which I would decide to become a Physician Assistant (PA). I thought to myself, If I can change a life, even just one, how many others will benefit as a result? Each decision we make has a ripple effect that changes not only our lives but also the lives of people around us.

Several years later I found myself stuck on the side of a very different cliff. My wife, who was 6 months pregnant, had developed bilateral pulmonary emboli (PE). It was uncommon for me to find her with tears in her eyes but one Sunday night she woke me up and while struggling to breath, told me that she couldn't lie down because her back hurt too much. Frightened and unsure what to do, I did my best to diagnose the problem. I had been trained as an EMT but that provided only a little help under such circumstances. I was suspicious that she had developed a PE but her legs showed no signs of deep vein thrombosis. We made the decision to visit the emergency department and after many hours and many tests, the diagnosis was confirmed and treatment began. It was exactly one week later that my wife called me from work with identical symptoms. At this point I had learned much more about PEs and according to the statistics, I became fairly certain I would soon have to say goodbye to my dear wife. I distinctly remember this terrible, wrenching feeling in my gut, the kind you get when your big brother punches you for being his little brother. Never in my life had I a wished that I could do more for a person than at that moment. I didn't have to say goodbye. The doctors and PAs changed her life. They took her from dying to living. They got her down from the cliff.

It certainly wasn't a light bulb moment. In fact, I had decided I wanted to be a PA almost a year prior. At the time I was the director of clinical research for a small industry research company. I worked with patients in nearly all therapeutic areas and together with our doctors and PAs we did our best to provide comfortable quality care to our patients as we investigated new medications. While my career was going well, I soon recognized that the part of my job I enjoyed most was the time I spent with my patients, conducting interviews, drawing blood, answering questions and providing education. I wanted more of that and while dodging traffic on the way to the ER, I realized that my desire to help my wife was a magnified version of what I had felt with all of my patients. Each interaction we have provides an opportunity for us to react and our reactions can change the lives of countless people even if we just start with one. Getting stuck on a cliff taught me that. I wanted desperately to finish Ha Ling Peak, but even more I wanted to be safe. I wanted a good professional career, but even more I want to treat and care for patients. I want to change lives. I want to take people from dying to living. I want to get them down from the cliff.

I never finished climbing Ha Ling Peak and finishing was probably never the point. Everyday there are limitless factors that are out of our control that will get us stuck on the cliff. Our job is to react and adapt to those changes in our circumstance. We are all shaped by moments, tiny portions of our everyday lives that form the majority of who we will become. I guess if you put these moments together you might call it experience. Whatever it's called, my moments have fixed in my mind a determined resolution to become PA.

Commentary Essay 31

You're a good writer, a huge plus, and have an excellent, easy to read yet sophisticated style. All those are sure to grab the attention of admissions folks. You've improved the essay since I last read it, but it still needs work.

You open with a literal cliff hanger, and I see that you're tied to the mountain climbing experience. The problem is that it doesn't work with the essay — it just doesn't fit in with the points you're making about wanting to be a PA. I think it's most apparent at the beginning and end of the essay which are general philosophical statements. You're straining to tie the climbing experience with your work/life experiences because you like it so much. (I understand — what a dramatic, scary, thrilling adventure). But if you are determined to open with the climbing experience, you need to re-think how you'll make it work thematically. Right now it's like reading about an apple in one sentence, about broccoli in the next. It's that disconnected.

Have a couple of friends or relatives read this part: "While in the uncomfortable embrace of disappointment and a climbing harness,

I had no idea that this moment would set the foundation on which I would decide to become a Physician Assistant (PA). I thought to myself, If I can change a life, even just one, how many others will benefit as a result? Each decision we make has a ripple effect that changes not only our lives but also the lives of people around us," and ask if they see how you get from the disappointment of leaving the mountain to wanting to change lives by becoming a PA.

The other issue is that you talk in depth about your wife's experience, but then say it wasn't a light bulb moment, that you'd already decided to be a PA. That undermines the whole episode (which by the way, is too long, although I was relieved to learn she survived).

Skip generalities. They don't help admissions folks know you, and that's what they're looking for. It's tempting to philosophize, but this essay is not the place.

You are on track when you start to talk about your work experiences, and when you talk about how the PAs and doctors impacted your wife's treatment. In those places you touch on why you want to be a PA. If you're going to use your wife's experience, focus more on the PA interactions and delete the beginning of the next paragraph. Otherwise, pick a patient that you treated and worked on with a PA.

Keep going. Writing is rewriting!

Essay 32

I anxiously walked through the doors and into the classroom where I would be helping teach Sunday school for a group of four-year old's. I looked around at all the children playing together and spotted one of the most beautiful girls I had ever seen. As she was running around the room waving a piece of paper, I went up to her and asked what her name was. There was no response she just kept running around with her piece of paper. I asked her name again, but she still did not respond. Her mother saw me trying to communicate with her and informed me that her name was Lily and that she was autistic and could not talk. My heart broke after hearing this, and I immediately wanted to do everything I could to help her. I listened intently as her mom showed me how to work with her, and I immediately fell in love. I ended up working with Lily for the next couple of years. It was difficult at times when people stared at us but it was worth seeing her smile and laugh.

While I did not recognize it at the time, Lily was one of the main reasons I decided to go into the medical field. I have had many other experiences, such as my mom's diagnosis of Multiple Sclerosis or my grandfather's Alzheimer's, but what makes Lily special, however, is that she gave me a new understanding of how to express love. Because she could not talk, she had to show her emotions through her actions. I knew by the way she would laugh uncontrollably while being spun around or by the way she would run up and give you a hug that she really did care. In the same way, I want to show my patients how important they are to me by listening to their needs and doing everything I can to help them. Lily also taught me that the first step to healing is love. Even as a high school student, I was able to help her just by loving her and showing her how much I cared. Through patience, love, and determination, I was able to watch Lily grow and accomplish many things. I knew whatever career I decided on, I wanted to experience that type of love.

Before working with Lily, I had never thought about being in the medical field. I did not know exactly what I wanted to do, but I knew that it had to involve helping others. Up until the end of my junior year of high school, I thought about going into forensics. I enjoyed watching NCIS and Criminal Minds and trying to solve the cases. I originally thought about being a police officer or working with the FBI, but I kept thinking about how much I loved working with Lily and decided to go into the medical field. I could not stand seeing others in pain and not knowing what to do to help them. Due to my athletic background, I originally thought about going into physical therapy. I intended to use these skills to work in the school system in order to continue working with children like Lily. However, after shadowing a PT, I felt as if there was something missing. I also want to do medical missions, and while a physical therapist would be able to help, I felt as if a PT would be limited in the services he could offer on the type of missions I want to do. It was not until I shadowed a physician assistant at St. Jude Children's Research Hospital that I felt the passion each doctor and physician assistant possessed towards every patient. In addition to treating each child, the physician assistant would take time to ask and check on the family that was staying with the patient. He knew how important the family was in order to help the child get better. I also loved how each patient was like trying to solve a case. The PA had to figure out what was causing the problem and then figure out how to fix it. I also loved the team atmosphere between the physician and the physician assistant. With multiple brains working together, I feel as if there is a higher chance of success.

I also considered going into research. After working for a semester in the Microbiology lab at Mississippi State University, however, I realized that one of the main components I loved about the physician assistant is the interaction he has with his patient. While I enjoyed my experience and discovering how the human body works, I want to be able to form relationships and directly take care of patients. Therefore, I believe that being a physician assistant is the right fit for me.

After deciding to go into the medical field, I tried getting as much medical experience as possible, which proved difficult because I was also a college cheerleader. Therefore, I shadowed and did internships, such as The Church Health Center and MDA camp, during all of my breaks. I finally decided not to cheer my senior year in order to obtain more medical experience. I feel, however, that the people skills and time management learned from cheering will help me when working with many different patients. I also feel that my strong academic background, as well as my passion for serving and helping others, will help make me a great physician assistant.

Commentary Essay 32

You have great heart, which comes through in your essay. But you don't want Admissions Directors to think that's all you have. Even though it sounds like you have quite a bit of experience from shadowing and internships, you haven't talked much about them.

The part about Lily is too long, and I'm afraid your focus on love sounds a little idealistic. (Even when you get past talking about Lily, you use "love" quite a bit — pick another word)! It's wonderful if that's what drives you, but it's not what will capture the attention of Admissions folks.

One of the things all Admissions faculty I interviewed said is they rather have patient/experience related information than family or personal experiences. Your interaction with Lily can be the start of your essay since she started you on the journey to becoming a PA, but limit it to one or two sentences. It sounds like that all happened while you were in high school. I know you've had a lot more experience with patients since that time by reading the rest of your essay. If I were editing your essay, the first two paragraphs would become one very short paragraph.

Rather than spending valuable space on what you don't want to do, like being a PT or researcher, consolidate those paragraphs into a sentence or two (omitting that you liked NCIS and Criminal Minds), and say more about what you learned while shadowing and interning. You can use a patient as an example to show what you learned about the profession and how that person enhanced your skills (if that applies) or made you realize you have skills that will help you be a good PA.

It's good that you talk about your strengths — your people skills, time management and compassion. You want people to know what you bring to the table.

You have good material! Your essay just needs consolidation of the less relevant topics and expansion of the more.

Essay 33

Pain. Suffering. Misery. The only thing worse than these things is not being able to do a single thing about them. My dad explained to me how my mom was very sick as he drove us to the hospital. I sat in silence and looked out the window. It was a calm autumn day and the leaves on the trees were an array of yellows and reds.

I walked through the intensive care unit; the sullen faces of family and friends looked down upon me. My body floated down the hallway towards her room. She lay on her hospital bed with several members of my family standing around her. They stepped back to let me see her as I walked up to her side, unsure of what to say or do. Her skin was yellow with jaundice and even little movements caused her great pain. When I opened my mouth to speak, I only broke down in tears.

Those next few weeks were the longest weeks of my life. Days stretched on as I went from school to the hospital to my home almost every day. Seeing my strong, independent mom struggle in the hospital upset and angered me deeply. I was frustrated by my inability to do anything of significance to cure her, so I did whatever simple tasks were needed of me.

When she was awake, I would sit next to her and comfort her. Whether I was simply holding her hand, telling her to be strong, or giving her water with an oral sponge, I did whatever I could. When the doctor would explain something to us, I did my best to understand what he was talking about. I would go home and look up what he said on the computer, only to be left with more questions. I wanted to know more and I wanted to be able to do more, but I couldn't and that was the hardest thing to accept. Her health was in the hospital's hands and I was left to wait and worry.

While working as a physical therapist aide, I always try to put myself in the patients' shoes and remember how I felt in the hospital with my mom. I really pay attention to what the therapist tells the patients so when they have those same questions, I will know the answer and can help them understand. This helps me learn more about the complex human body and it helps quell any concerns the patients may have. I love being able to give them tips and ideas on how to feel better, even if it's something as simple as telling them to put a pillow between their legs while they sleep to alleviate back pain and help them get a better night's rest. If my little piece of advice can result in them being happier and in less pain, then I know those long ten-hour days were worth it.

During our short time on Earth, we strive to find a purpose for our existence. We experiment and search for a passion that motivates us to work harder and be better. Sitting at my mom's bedside in the hospital, I discovered my passion. Being a physical therapy aide allows me to make use of my passion, but there is still so much I can't do. When the patients come in, I can't be the one to stretch them and massage them. As a physician assistant, I can be sure that each patient gets the care they need and deserve because I will be one of the providers giving it. I can do everything in my power to educate them and help them be as healthy as they can be.

My ultimate goal is to be a physician assistant in orthopedic surgery. The complexities of the human musculoskeletal system have always been of curiosity to me and working in physical therapy has only enhanced that interest. Working alongside a physician in orthopedics, I will have that ability to help rid patients of their pain, their suffering, and their misery.

Commentary Essay 33

You're a very good writer. Your descriptions have complexity and depth. (There's a bit of drama that you don't need — your body didn't float down a hall, for example. Things like that are distracting).

While the sections about your mother are done well, you spend too much time on them. Every Admissions person I interviewed said to focus on your adult experiences. A couple of sentences about your early experience can be your opening. Then move into your work.

You've developed good skills — compassion, paying attention to detail and listening among them. Expand on those using a patient as an example if it helps explain. Instead of saying what you can't do, talk about what you've learned from your job and how that will make you a good PA.

You'll need to beef up the part that leads to why you want to be a PA. If you've shadowed or worked with a PA, talk about it.

Essay 34

November 6th, 2010, *********, New York in my aunt's red GMC Acadia with her, my mom, grandmother and cousin around 5:00pm; this was the moment that I was told my mom had been diagnosed with breast cancer. They had all driven to visit me at ********* University for dinner and to tell me the news. I had never been so scared in my life. As a child of divorced parents, with an essentially nonexistent father, seeing the potential to lose my mother shattered my world.

November 26th, 2010, ********, New York, in the living room of my grandmother's house with my mom, grandmother, and grandfather at approximately 3:00pm; this was the moment that my aunt called to tell us she had just been diagnosed with breast cancer. Now I could clearly see the possibility that, along with my mom, my aunt could also be taken away. I literally fell to my knees and begged God for their lives.

My love for science began in the fourth grade, but those two moments along with the following months and years of surgeries, doctor's appointments, and physical and emotional healing secured my ambition to practice medicine. I suddenly found it immensely important to attend every doctor's appointment, getting rides from whomever was available between school and home, taking notes, and doing as much research as possible to help my family understand and make the best decisions they could. Being able to do that gave me the opportunity to show them how much I care, and I found that caring for them completely fulfilled me.

At the time, I hadn't realized how impactful the situation was. I found myself overwhelmed between classes, work, volunteering, friends, and helping my family every chance I could and I began to fail all around. Grades began to drop, volunteering was cut short, and stress skyrocketed. Looking back I can honestly say I had never had so many responsibilities and commitments before and therefore severely lacked time management and prioritization skills I so desperately needed. After seeing my lowest grades of all time during my sophomore year and realizing how I had fallen in love with helping and caring for others through my family's situation and volunteer experience, I gained a sense of motivation unlike any I'd had before. Through determination, recently learned time management skills, and help from classmates and professors, I was able to bring my grades back up and make dean's list once again.

That same year, my guidance counselor, professor, and one of the most knowledgeable persons I have known to date, Dr. ****, who knew my desire to work in medicine, suggested I look into the Physician Assistant profession. After doing very little research, I decided that was not the career for me I am someone who wants to be my own boss or so I thought.

Less than a year later, in October of 2012 I was parked at a 7/11 convenience store in ******** waiting for one of my best friends, when I saw a gold Chevy Tahoe lose control going about 50 MPH and begin rolling down the road, into the oncoming lane, cross the oncoming lane, and come to a stop in a restaurant parking lot after hitting a light pole. With out even thinking I turned my car off, stepped out and ran to the road. That was when I realized aside from CPR I had no knowledge of what to do to help any of the people that may be in that car. I began to run back to my car to grab my cell phone and call the Police, when I saw an ambulance parked at the gas station next door to the 7/11. Shaking from my emotions, almost in tears, and slightly out of breath, I ran to the paramedics and explained what I witnessed. They immediately called in the accident and drove away with sirens screaming and lights flashing.

I went back to my car with the largest sense of relief. The people in that car would be helped in the correct way and the best way that those trained paramedics could offer, which was much greater than what I could offer. That experience helped me realized that having a professional that is willing to help you and offer a greater deal of experience, knowledge, and wisdom would be a blessing not a lack of knowledge or independence. I found that learning more about medicine and treatment by those who have much more knowledge and experience than I is what I look forward to most.

After graduation from college, with a renewed motivation to become a physician assistant, I found two jobs as a caregiver and nurses assistant. The first job at Comfort Keepers requires that I go into other peoples homes and help their loved ones by offering a variety of services ranging from companionship and cooking meals to monitoring blood pressure, heart rate, blood oxygen levels, medication reminders, incontinence care, and bathing. The second job is in the dementia care unit at Belmont

Village Senior Living Center where we focused much more on feeding, incontinence care, bathing, medication reminders, and closely monitoring and reporting each residents' mental and physical status and deterioration due to Alzheimer's and Dementia. The jobs became the ultimate test of my patience and desire to work in medicine. But ultimately I found them completely rewarding and humbling. At the end of the day, I can say that I have helped someone perform some vital activities that made it possible for him or her to get through the day. I have formed friendships with many of my coworkers and patients. These caregivers and family's demonstrate an enormous amount of compassion and humanity for those they are caring for and it is the most inspired I have felt. Those coworkers, who have chosen that career path because they love helping these elderly patients, no matter how difficult the job may be, especially humble and inspire me.

I have done much more research and have consulted with all the medical doctors, physician assistants, nurses, and professors I know, and I realize now that this was the exact career I have been dreaming of since the 4th grade. Becoming a physician assistant encompasses everything I love: science, medicine, helping others, continual learning, and a degree of independence in the workplace. This career path is the fulfillment of my dreams. Armed with the knowledge and experience I have gained through my past experiences, struggles and shortcomings, I know there is nothing that will deter me from accomplishing this dream and I am willing and eager to prove it.

**** specifics are omitted for privacy.

Commentary Essay 34

This is an excellent start to what will be a great essay. Your writing skills are good — I saw few grammar errors.

The main problem is that you spend too much time on family/personal experiences and not enough on your healthcare related experiences. It's important to explain why your grades dropped and you did a great job on that. Shorten those first few paragraphs so you can focus on what's important to Admissions personnel.

I would never say in an essay that you did not want to be a PA, even though you later changed your mind. If I were a reader, I might stop right there.

Use some of your experiences with a specific patient or two to demonstrate your skills. You say you have patience, compassion, an interest in continual learning — show it with details. You need to paint the picture to make your essay come alive.

You don't say why you decided to become a PA instead of another healthcare professional. Admissions folks want to know what specifically appeals to you about the profession and why you'd make a good PA. Have you worked with PAs? Shadowed any? Talk about those experiences.

Essay 35

I had never seen someone so frightened in my life. "Excuse me, Ms. Lewis," I said. "Ms. Lewis! We're ready for you now." Her husband helped her to her feet as I came over with a wheelchair. I helped her sit down and wheeled her out of the waiting area. She looked over her shoulder to her husband and I could see her eyes welling with tears. I asked her if everything was okay or if she felt faint. She nodded and said that she was fine in a shaky voice. She told me that she has never had surgery before and that this would be her first time. I assured her that our staff would do everything we could to make sure that she does well and recovers soon. I told her that the surgeons at our hospital were excellent and would do everything in their power to help her. I told her that our nurses would be there to make sure that she was comfortable and well taken care of. She uttered a thank you as I wheeled her to the Nurse's Station. I told her that Nurse Black would be her nurse for the day and that she was an excellent nurse. I then wheeled her to her room and helped her out of the wheelchair. I told her again that everything would be fine. Her surgeon, Dr. White, came in and greeted everyone. I directed him to Ms. Lewis' room and went back to the Nurse's Station for chart preparation and discharge instructions. An hour or so had passed and Ms. Lewis returned from surgery. Soon it was time to discharge her so that she could go home. I loaded her back into the wheelchair and we continued to talk. She thanked me again, saying that my words made her feel a little better about her procedure. She told me to thank the nurses and the doctors for everything that they did for her. I had been a volunteer for some time now and while I play a minor, almost forgettable, part on the floor of the One Day Surgery, people still give me an emphatic "thank you" for what I do for them.

I initially wanted to volunteer because love for medicine and helping people reawakened after I survived the April 27, 2011 tornado. There was a call to action where everybody who could help came out to help whenever they had availability. Initially, I worked at the hub station the American Red Cross set up in my neighborhood. While I was not a healthcare professional, I could volunteer and offer my services in other ways. The extent of this was signing people up for services so that they could go into the hub station to get vouchers for food, clothes, toys, or anything else they needed.

In May of 2011, I graduated from a small college in Birmingham, Alabama. I knew I wanted to work in the medical field, but was not sure of the exact profession I wanted to pursue. I spoke with the volunteer coordinator at a local hospital and she was happy to have me come volunteer with her program. I created great relationships with the healthcare professionals at the hospital during my time as a volunteer. I spoke with nurses about their jobs, school, how they handle patients, and I even saw first hand how they interacted with the patients. I spoke to doctors about tests, schools, their workload, how they coped with things, and their patient interactions.

I surveyed Patient Care Techs, Med Techs, CRNA's, and everybody in between just to get a feel of what it is I really wanted to do. Everybody was interested in my decision and offered me advice every time they saw me. I have the utmost respect for all healthcare professionals and I appreciate them for what they do for the community. However, when deciding what profession would be best for me, the physicians and P.A.'s resonated with me the most. I also attended an informational about the Physician Assistant program and feel in love. It is not about the status or the superficial power of being in charge. It is about having the influence to make someone better, knowing what to do in order to cure diseases, and even preventing the diseases all together.

Knowing that I can make a difference in someone's life or influence him or her is worth more than money or any other kind of repayment. The summer I volunteered was one of my most memorable and most fulfilling moments to date. This solidified my thoughts that the healthcare field is something that I wanted to strive to work in and achieve. When I think back to my time as a volunteer, people like Ms Lewis come to mind. With me (in my head), doing so little, making such an impact on her (and others like her) makes me want to put myself in a position so that I can do even more. If allowed to be a part of the Physician Assistant program I would be extremely thankful but also extremely determined to make everybody happy who has placed their faith in me to do better and become something better. I know that I can be a great Physician Assistant if given the opportunity.

Commentary Essay 35

First of all, this is not terrible! You've had some unique experiences which will give you a great basis to build on.

To start, shorten the first paragraph. It's a good place to open, but way too long.

It sounds like you haven't had much hands on health care related experience from what you've written. If that's the case, then you'll use your volunteer work to demonstrate how you've built your skills over time. Instead of telling how you spoke with professionals about different fields of medicine, show that you know how they did their jobs, what you learned from watching them, and why those experiences led to the decision to apply to PA school. You never mentioned that you worked with PAs. If you came across PAs in your volunteer work, talk about what you learned, what impressed you, and why PAs stand apart from others.

Your goal is to convince schools that you know exactly what a PA does, that your skills match those needed to be a PA (I'm not talking about clinical skills since you don't have them, I'm talking about things like patience, empathy, an inquisitive mind, attention to detail — all the things that make a good PA).

There are a few grammar errors in your essay. It would be a good idea to have people read your essay to correct those.

Essay 36

Out trekking we made a short stop in a village near the Laos China border. A man, Noy, had been in a serious motorcycle accident. The closest clinic was over 100 miles away and he had no desire to make the trip. His leg was in pieces with several open, bright red wounds. There was no cast, no pain medication, only herbal Chinese medicine that smelled of vinegar and rotting flesh. My first aid class was enough to know he had two choices: get to a hospital or stay home and let the infection continue, leading to amputation or death. He chose to stay home.

I still don't know what happened to Noy. We were sent on our way, told that the village would take care of him. We spent three days trekking in Northern Laos, speaking often of him and asking ourselves if, as outsiders, we should have done something different, potentially life saving. The next few nights, I incessantly asked myself, 'Why have I spent three years managing a restaurant in Laos when I could have been doing more, meeting a true need?'

Two weeks later, I learned for the first time what a Physician Assistant (PA) was while eating lunch with a doctor, asking about her decision to enter medicine. At 30 years old, married and without children, I was unwilling to spend 8-10 years in school. As she explained that a PA ran the clinic at the US embassy in Laos, I knew then what I wanted to be.

The past year volunteering in an ED and shadowing a MD and his PAs has confirmed what I believed after researching the profession; that is, it fits perfectly with what I want to do. I will provide personalized, compassionate medical care as an integral part of a team for disadvantaged people like Noy. While managing a café in Laos, I learned the importance of empowering others and that a team united achieves most. As an English teacher in Ho Chi Minh City, Vietnam, I discovered how important it is to connect personally with each student and that cookie cutter explanations are lazy. The last year and a half in school and my job as a science tutor have convinced me that the difference between an A and a B is merely the amount of time and work put in. These qualities are also what I see most often when shadowing great PAs. York College provides a unique, diverse atmosphere that is best suited for my life experiences and who I want to become.

Perhaps Noy is healthy and back on his motorcycle. Maybe he isn't. What I know is I want to be able to give back to people like him. I also know I don't have to travel back to Laos to do so. I am excited to start the journey to becoming a PA and ask if you would be willing to instruct me in what it takes to change lives like Noy's.

Commentary Essay 36

This essays does a great job of fitting a lot of information into a very short yet cohesive statement.

Still, I'd change a few things. Some are minor, some bigger.

A minor suggestion — instead of using the words "bright red," I'd say "bloody." It's more descriptive and accurate.

The third paragraph needs work. You definitely don't want to make it sound that you picked PA school because it wouldn't be as much work or time as medical school, which is what it sounds like. Your friend's description likely piqued your interest, but I doubt you decided you wanted to be a PA on the spot. That doesn't sound real to me.

Essay 37

Every experience life throws at you bears significance in how it shapes you as a person. A lot of people take their experiences for granted as they do not truly understand the significance it holds in their life. As one grows older and wiser, reflection begins to occur and that is when direction is brought into life.

The experience that began it all consisted of a grimace of pain spread across her face as she cried with every move her body made. A middle-aged woman laid on the bed in front of me slowly passing away from uterine cancer. Everyone moved strategically as a team while providing her care. While looking in her eyes and knowing she was receiving quality care in ensuring her comfort, the need for compassion was seen. I immediately put my hand on hers as we were completing her treatment and assured her that her family was coming. I could see a sense of peace come over her as her family walked into the room to spend their final moments together. In this moment I knew that I wanted to work in a healthcare team with people providing quality care while showing compassion.

The next influential experience began in a small crowded Nicaraguan schoolroom having no windows where I sat with a middle aged man named Arturo whose face demonstrated decades of hard work and wear. He came at the opportunity for receiving free health treatment provided by the Joining Education Through Service group I had been a part of. An initial observation of his health showed no major concerns besides existing diabetes and complications related to it. That was until he described pain in his foot, which resulted in him revealing a wound exposing the bone on his foot once the bandages came off due to him not taking care of his health conditions appropriately, Additional medical professionals were immediately called to my aid and after an evaluation of the wound was done, it was determined that Arturo had to immediately go to the hospital at the risk of having to amputate his foot. While waiting, I proceeded to educate the man on diabetes and management of the disease in order to improve his understanding and ability to better care for his condition. In this moment I further was affirmed that I wanted to work within a team, showing compassion and treating patients with quality care, while educating them on how to improve their health.

As I continued in my journey I found myself always being drawn to the Physician Assistant who works among others seamlessly in a team, but always demonstrates autonomy as well. I was first able to witness this as I volunteered in hospitals and had the opportunity to learn about various health professions where I saw how each member worked in their role within the hospital setting. I further had the opportunity to see this role through healthcare shadowing. The PA was always a leader, but also worked in the team as a leading supporter which was what I had found as being critical to me in my future career. During my experience shadowing with a neurology and neurosurgery PA, I saw a leader that treated numerous patients in the clinic setting but I also saw the leading supporter within the surgery room working together with the physician through the process of a vagus nerve stimulation and lumbar microdiscectomy.

The final experience providing me direction came as I had the opportunity to really look at illness in an objective view. A small frail woman named Sherry truly taught me the meaning of that. "I can't" Sherry had told me one day as she looked me in the eyes with despair. Although she did not specify what she meant when she spoke those words I immediately knew that she felt powerless laying trapped in her little frame. Her strength was diminishing before her eyes and her ability to care for herself independently continually decreased. Seeing Sherry on an almost daily basis the toll could be seen in her face and the power of compassion and true care was a necessity. Every work day, taking the extra time with Sherry was my necessity. Addressing her concerns, discussing her goals, and encouraging motivation to work towards recovery allowed me to see what she was lacking. Someone to listen and take the time to provide her with quality care.

 Through Sherry I also had realized that challenges always arise and are meaningful in the sense that they allow us to better ourselves, such as I have experienced through challenging courses in my undergraduate career. As I experienced difficulty in subject matter I grew from these challenges in order to better myself through improving my knowledge of the subject matter within receiving tutoring within the subject as well as eventually providing tutoring in order to continue improving and fine tuning my own knowledge base.

There are many attributes of a PA that I admire and would like to fulfill. I have a desire for learning and teaching others, which I have demonstrated through tutoring in many different subject matters, and through my work and volunteer experiences in which I was able to educate others on various health matters. I feel this is congruent with an important attribute of being a PA as you are lifelong learners that continually grow in knowledge within the field and educate those that are being served.

Commentary Essay 37

Before I forget, there a few grammar issues:

- Never capitalize "physician assistant" unless it's part of a formal name.

- A comma goes after the last word in dialog ("I can't," Sherry had told me).

- You have a comma where there should be a period (. . . appropriately. Additional . . .)

- In one place you had two periods. (career..)

It's hard to edit our own work, so be sure to have someone take a fresh look at it before you turn it in. Those types of mistakes are not taken lightly by Admissions Directors and faculty. Carelessness is not a good trait for a PA!

That being said, I like the idea you open with — that every experience shapes us. It's a good opening sentence and I would leave it. But the rest of the paragraph can go. For one you never really say anything more about not recognizing the significance of an experience. The third is a different way of saying the second sentence, and is so general, it doesn't add anything. The opening is a general statement, and if you're going to make a broad, philosophical statement, it needs to tie in to the essay itself. Admissions Directors and faculty have said they don't generally like them, and I understand why — they aren't personal to the writer.

In the second paragraph, the first sentence needs more of a transition. It should read something like: "The experience that began my journey to becoming a PA . . . ."

The two examples of inciting experiences are great, because they have different lessons. Excellent job on that.

Overall, your essay is a little wordy. Look for places where you can cut. One of those places is the conclusion. The last sentence in particular, is wordy without making a strong point. Read the entire essay carefully and be merciless with the delete key. Remember, Admissions folks literally read thousands of essays in a session.

One final thing — your conclusion doesn't really tie your essay together. It's more along the lines of your fourth paragraph. Basically, it talks about another part of being a PA — the fact that PAs educate. You can weave that information in elsewhere and write a strong conclusion to wrap up your essay.

Remember, writing is rewriting! Once you fix these relatively minor issues, you'll have a great essay.

Essay 38

It was my junior year of high school and I was preparing to apply to the New Visions Medical Career Program. A few months had passed and finally a letter had come; I was accepted into this rigorous, hands on program. From the first day we were immersed into the bustling hospital setting, interacting with medical professionals and patients with various diagnoses and issues. On my assigned weeklong rotation with a primary care physician, he said to me "I may not know every detail about each of my patients, but I know their faces and a little something about them."

I thought to myself, this is exactly how I want to interact with my patients when I become a doctor. These experiences inspired my journey and aspirations.

A year later, I found myself sitting at a presentation held by the U**** premedical club, listening to a physician assistant describing her career and its benefits. I was struck by her enthusiasm. It then occurred to me that I did not have to be in school for several years and commit to one specialty to be the practitioner I aspired to be. I realized then that pursuing a career as a PA would afford me more social freedoms while simultaneously allowing me to have the option to practice a variety of medical specialties. I started to take classes that were required prerequisites for PA school. This is also when I decided to take the EMT class that was offered on campus, although I was already taking 17 credits; this is what I wanted to do, and has been one of the best decisions I have made thus far. Upon obtaining my certification I joined a local ambulance agency. There I volunteered as much as possible. I would go in on my own time for 5, 8, 10 hour shifts. Sometimes there were no calls that day, but I would read previous charts and practice my skills. I soaked up as much as I could.

After receiving mostly simple and basic calls, we were dispatched to a cardiac arrest. Upon arrival on scene I was directed by the paramedic to administer respirations with a bag valve mask. Focusing on the patient's face and hearing a loved one in the background, I realized that this job was not going to be easy, but I knew it was my responsibility and his life was in my hands.

It is so interesting to link my clinical experience to my coursework at school. I have had several patients complaining of chest pain, and when the paramedic conducts an EKG and says the patient has an abnormal T wave or a left bundle branch block, I never really knew what that meant. Recently, while reading about the cardiovascular system in anatomy and physiology, I found myself recalling these patients and now understanding their condition. I am realizing more and more that my innate sense of care and compassion, combined with my demanding coursework will make me an excellent, well rounded PA for the benefit of my patients.

Being a physician assistant means providing the patient with the best care possible, regardless of other factors. As a PA I will ensure that my patients are knowledgeable of their illness and all of the treatment options. I will ensure that my patients are able to receive the best treatments and will be sympathetic to their needs. I know that I will be put into difficult situations and I am prepared to use the knowledge I have accumulated to treat my patient at the optimal level.

Commentary Essay 38

Your essay is concise and to the point, which is excellent. And your first paragraph is well done.

If I were Admissions Directors, I'd probably stop reading when I got the part where you say you want to be a PA because it will give you more social freedoms and require less schooling than medical school. They're looking for people who aspire to be a PA because they love the profession, and are motivated to work hard to achieve excellence. So focus on things that PAs do that appeal to you. For example, you briefly mention that as a PA you'll have the ability to work in a variety of fields. PAs are often more connected to their patients than the physicians — you've already mentioned the importance of the doctor/patient relationship in the first paragraph. That seems meaningful to you, so tell about it.

You have a great opportunity to actually link your coursework to your experience by using an interaction with a patient as an example. You almost do it, but not quite. Right now in the essay they're more parallel than connected.

There are some generalizations I'd edit out, like "regardless of other factors." When you only have a limited number of characters, you'll want every word to count.

The bones of your essay are good. Now you need to flesh it out to make it come alive.

Essay 39

"To say I was an accident prone child is an understatement. I frequented doctors' offices and emergency rooms for a variety of injuries and ailments. I remember staying home sick from elementary school, curling up on the sofa to watch marathons of "Medical Mysteries" and "Trauma: Life in the ER". My squeamish parents were somewhat disgusted by my gruesome choice of entertainment and were puzzled by my infatuation with medicine. Even so, my interest and enthusiasm for medical care persisted.

In 2006, after I was involved in a serious golf cart accident, I knew for certain that I would pursue a career in healthcare. I suffered extensive injuries after being ejected from the vehicle, run over, and dragged along the pavement. I remember the rushed atmosphere and commotion of the emergency room as I lay there feeling shocked by the gravity of the situation. Then,

Michelle walked in, a smiling brunette clad in a crisp white coat. I assumed she was a physician as she explained the imaging procedures and tests I would soon undergo. She addressed me not as a naïve thirteen-year-old but simply as a concerned patient. She answered all my questions and stayed engaged in our conversation even as she performed an intraarticular injection to determine if my knee joint had been compromised. I was in awe at the combination of her technical proficiency and calm disposition. Not until years later, after attending a physician assistant symposium in college, did I realize Michelle was a physician assistant.

After my accident, my passion for medicine persisted. In high school, I enrolled in Honors Anatomy and Physiology and was fascinated by the field trips to watch an open-heart surgery and visit a cadaver lab. My teachers noted my enthusiasm for the subject and nominated me to attend a medical leadership conference at Georgetown University. When selecting a college major, I chose Nutritional Sciences because of the strong focus on biological science; it also provided a unique perspective on clinical work and emphasized the critical thinking skills necessary in practice. I worked assiduously because I knew exemplary academics were necessary when applying to graduate programs. However, despite struggling with a personal crisis during my sophomore year, I was determined not to let one semester mar the academic record I had worked so hard to achieve. I made significant changes in my life and learned how to maximize my academic potential while managing stress in a healthy way. This experience was a critical point of self-exploration, and I am confident it was an important step in preparing me for the rigors of PA school.

Once I was comfortable managing the challenges of a science heavy course load, I began to focus on gaining more experience working in healthcare. Although my interest to learn the intricacies of medicine was undeniable, I was still unsure about which career would be the best fit for me. I spoke with doctors, nurses, and PAs to determine the differences between these types of practitioners. While trying to make a decision, I repeatedly thought of Michelle, my earliest inspiration. I saw clearly that compared to other healthcare professionals, PAs have a unique opportunity to build a rapport with their patients by getting to know them on a personal level, which is what I value most.

However, it was not until I became a certified nursing assistant at an assisted living facility that I truly understood how much I valued being a part of someone's healing process. Initially, I saw the job as an opportunity to work collaboratively with other healthcare professionals, but I realized quickly the magnitude of this experience was much greater than I anticipated. It is remarkable to watch the aging process unfold and see the devastating progression of diseases. It is my responsibility to not only provide care to the residents, but also to be vigilant about changes in their condition, to be compassionate about the struggles they endure in light of their impending mortality, and to listen to them when nobody else will. These moments make me realize what an honor it is to be a healthcare provider.

Although my academic journey has always been aimed towards a career in medicine, my unique life experiences are what inspired me to become a physician assistant. The PA profession encompasses my passion for scientific knowledge and my desire to build relationships with patients. Pursuing such a fulfilling and exciting career leaves me with a profound sense of purpose and the definitive notion I will be a successful physician assistant.

Commentary Essay 39

I like the image of you as a kid watching medical shows on TV, but for purposes of this essay, you're taking up valuable space that could be used to talk about your healthcare experiences in more detail. When I interviewed Admissions Directors and faculty from across the country, every person said they weren't interested in hearing childhood experiences. I'd delete the entire first paragraph of your essay.

Your second paragraph is good (skip the brunette in your description of Michelle — it's a wasted word).

The third paragraph needs editing — it reads well, but it has extra verbiage that has little significance. Remember, the people reading your essay are literally reading more than a thousand so save words where you can. And the word passion is so overused, it's meaningless. I rarely recommend using it. This is what I'd do in an edit:

"My interest in medicine persisted. When selecting a college major, I chose Nutritional Sciences because of the strong focus on biological science; it also provided a unique perspective on clinical work and emphasized the critical thinking skills necessary in practice. Despite struggling with a personal crisis during my sophomore year, I was determined not to let one semester mar the academic record I had worked so hard to achieve. I made significant changes and learned how to manage stress in a healthy way. This experience was a critical point of self-exploration, and I am confident it was an important step in preparing me for the rigors of PA school."

Use the extra space to elaborate a bit more on why you're choosing to be a PA as opposed to any other health care professional.

Essay 40

A nurse peeked through the door of the waiting room – "okay John, come on back." I looked up at my fiancé as he waddled toward the door in pain, and I followed closely behind. Several months ago a dermatologist had diagnosed him with Hidradenitis suppurativa (HS), an idiopathic autoimmune skin condition that resulted in chronic episodes and remissions of painful cysts all over the body. This time it had attacked his tailbone.

As we waited in the exam room and the nurse collected vitals and history, I already had a scenario predetermined in my head: after reading the nurses notes, the doctor would come in, look at the cyst briefly, state that we'd have to drain it, and leave to prepare all within 60 seconds. However what happened next didn't fit my script. After the nurse left, a smiling young man came in and introduced himself as Todd, a Physician Assistant (PA). He sat down with us, inquired about history, pain and John's frustrations with the condition. He displayed a significant familiarity with this obscure disease. Finally when he examined the cyst, he did agree that we needed to drain it, but then sat down again and explained exactly the procedure he'd complete. The explanation was well appreciated by both of us, since John is deathly afraid of even minor surgeries, mostly because of the needles involved for local anesthetic. Even more appreciated was the patience and empathy he showed during the procedure, despite John's anger and anxiety as soon as the needle came out. When the ordeal was over and the wound neatly packed, Todd was still warm and friendly as he gave us our discharge instructions and wished us on our way. John and I both thanked him, grateful for his compassion.

That was my first encounter with a PA. Since middle school I'd been fascinated with clinical work, probably as a result of spending many days in the back of my dad's dental clinic as a kid. I had no interest specifically in dentistry, but I loved the clinical environment and the idea of helping people heal and remain healthy. Knowing the level of achievement necessary for getting into medical school, I had always kept school as a priority, even through my somewhat troubled teenage years. In fact I was studying for the MCAT that day in the waiting room, about to be a senior at Fort Lewis College. But the interaction with Todd, who was no doubt an amazing provider, had me curious about the PA profession and sparked a long period of investigation.

Several months of research, shadowing and interviews later, I had realized why becoming a PA was the perfect fit for me. I am fascinated and excited about the development of the Physician Assistant model. The idea of working as a team to improve patient care is brilliant, and this really appeals to me because I have always favored the idea of being a fundamental member of an effective team over the idea of working alone. No one person can ever know everything, and having multiple providers not only improves efficiency, but betters the quality of care with a system of checks and balances to avoid error and ensure that treatment plans are tailored to each patient. The fact that PAs can often achieve an advanced level of autonomy and are tasked with doing routine physical exams, diagnosing, followups, pre and postoperative care and even oversee their own set of patients is also appealing to me. I would likely be able to spend more time with each patient, but still address acute issues when necessary. Then when encountering a more complex case, I can always refer to my supervising physician for help. To me, this is the ideal balance of autonomy and assistance.

Finally, perhaps one of the most attractive factors about the PA profession is the ability to gain experience in a myriad of different fields. I always hated the idea of having to limit myself to only one area of medicine by choosing a residency. I would love to be open to work in almost any field and become competent in several specialties within my career. I may even be able to start out in a high workload field in my younger years, such as emergency medicine or surgery, but be able to switch to a lower intensity area like an outpatient clinic as I get older. My interests are far too broad to embrace the idea of being in the same field for my entire life. I am and will always be someone who thrives on learning new information. To be able to practice within many areas and gain as much medical knowledge as possible would be, for me, the ultimate satisfaction.

I truly believe that I have what it takes to become a skilled and compassionate PA. Everything about the profession seems perfectly tailored to my desires as a future clinician, and I can't wait to begin on this career path. I hope that you will consider me for your highly competitive program, and if you do I can promise that I will not disappoint.

Commentary Essay 40

Before I forget, be sure to use proper grammar. For example, write, "Okay, come on back, John." instead of, "okay John, come on back." Also, don't use contractions in these essays. The bottom line is that grammar errors will count against you.

Your essay has good bones. I like the opening (although I'd probably use a different word than "waddle." It has a negative connotation, and you could leave out the word, "okay"). You explain why you're interested in becoming a PA, which is also good.

The main problem is that you haven't told the Admissions folks anything about yourself that would make them interested in you as a candidate. Shorten the paragraphs about John and Todd to three or four sentences, and write about your shadowing experiences. What did you learn about yourself? Do you possess some similar skills/traits to those of the PA? I'm not talking about clinical skills, but rather leadership, patience, etc. Were you able to do anything except watch? If so, write about what you did, even it was to smile or hold someone's hand.

Don't waste space speculating on your career trajectory, and be careful about just telling what PAs do without tying it to your experiences. You could cut most of the third paragraph including this: "Then when encountering a more complex case, I can always refer to my supervising physician for help." I'd recommend starting fresh with that paragraph.

Have you done anything that requires team work? Have you volunteered anywhere? If you have write about it. Perhaps you've developed leadership skills that will help you as a PA. Are you a self-starter? What experiences could illustrate that?

Your conclusion talks about your compassion and skills. If that's your conclusion, they'll need to show up in the body of the essay. I'm sure you have them or you wouldn't be interested in being a PA.

Make your paragraphs shorter and separate them with a space — you want to make it easy for your reader to pay attention. Remember, they're reading over 1,000 essays.

I hope this helps. Remember, writing is rewriting!

Essay 41

She's a nightmare to work with," he muttered as he came out of her room. "That's why I refuse to work with her," another one of my coworkers stated. Jane was famously one of our most demanding residents. She liked everything a particular way, lacked patience, and assumed we could read her mind. The first couple of weeks that I worked with her I was emotionally and physically exhausted each time I left her room, my own patience stretched to its thinnest. It seemed like no matter how hard I tried I just could not connect with her. Then one day, as I was working hard to remember her routine for getting into bed—one flat pillow under each leg with the open side down, the seams of the sheets folded outward, her shoes tucked side by side under her dresser—I realized she was no longer barking orders at me. Instead, she was quietly examining a book with pictures of cats while I worked. As I was finishing up, she said "I love cats. This book here has such beautiful ones. Will you read the little lines of text at the bottom of each page for me?" When I nodded and took the book from her, I saw her smile for the first time since I began working at that facility. And our connection continued to grow stronger. After listening intently to her preferences, I was able to anticipate that flipping the pillow over to the cooler side would make her feel better or that she needed fresh coffee in her favorite cup. She smiled every time I work with her and even called me her "angel." She also became more cooperative, refusing showers less frequently and learning to speak her mind in a kinder manner. It amazed me how her attitude transformed after we had connected on a personal level.

In this day and age of amazing technological advances, with hundreds of ways to connect to other people, it is impressive how often face-to-face communication is abandoned. We forget how crucial that connection is to build trust, or any type of positive relationship. This is especially important in the medical field, as patients will surely feel lost and fearful without a trusting relationship with their health care providers. While working as a CNA in a longterm care facility, building positive relationships with the residents, like Jane, was imperative for their participation in their activities of daily living and cooperation with us as CNAs, nurses, CMAs, physical therapists, dietitians, physician assistants and doctors.

Through various experiences, it has become clear to me that forming connections is vital in the process of helping others. In college I coordinated and tutored for a program called Tutors for a Cause. We, as enthusiastic college students, were excited to be able to give back to our community by tutoring and mentoring elementary, middle and high school students who were also children and grandchildren of the college dining hall and maintenance staff. However, becoming a good tutor and mentor did not happen overnight. It took a lot of effort to really connect with the kids. In order to get them excited about learning, we had to think creatively and work as a team. One day we did a fun interactive presentation about gases, involving a hardboiled egg getting sucked into a seemingly too small glass bottle. The kids loved it. It sparked a general interest in physics and chemistry, even among some of the most apathetic students. After a couple more fun science experiments, the field trip at the end of the semester ended up being to a science museum, by request of the kids.

At an accessible and affordable medical clinic in rural Ecuador, quickly connecting with the patients was crucial for making them comfortable. While the doctor and nurse were busy wrapping up with the preceding patient, my job was to welcome the new patients and take their vitals. Whether it was an elderly woman, a young man, a screaming baby and her anxious mother, each and every patient was nervous about their impending procedure or exam. As I gained experience, I quickly learned how to speak confidently yet kindly and comfortingly in Spanish with each patient. These positive interactions with the patients upon their arrival made their brief time with us less difficult.

These experiences have helped me understand that I am meant to work with and try to help people. I have discovered that even the smallest degree of personal connection can make a difference in someone's life. Physician assistants perform valuable work and form personal connections with patients. This is the ideal way for me to use my strong work ethic and enthusiasm to work alongside patients and other members of the medical team. Together we can work to form connections, leading to trust and cooperation, and eventually a more positive health care experience.

Commentary Essay 41

Good start! You've outlined many of your experiences and connected them to lessons you learned as a result.

That's not to say your essay doesn't need editing. (Sorry). Grammar first. We don't know who "he" is, so write, "My coworker at (the type of facility). You don't need the other quote because you write that Jane was famously one of your most demanding patients.

You can shorten the paragraph about Jane. Same with the tutoring one. They both go on too long and in too much detail. More importantly, they both end with the same point — that you have the ability to make personal connections. That's also the same message I got from your Ecuador experience. (By the way, tell if it was volunteer work or paid).

The main message I took from your essay is that you have patience and can connect with your patients. Highlight others skills, such as leadership, team work, etc. You touch on those in your tutoring section, but not enough. You need to expand on those because being compassionate isn't enough.

You also haven't said why you want to be a PA as opposed to a CNA, nurse or doctor. Have you worked with PAs? Shadowed? What skills/traits do you have that mirrors theirs? What about the profession appeals to you and why?

Essay 42

Beige walls and black furniture made the waiting room seem like a spread in a home magazine. Pictures of sweeping landscapes replaced those of cartoons while the noise of a water feature substituted children playing. "Chelsea." A lady dressed in pink floral scrubs emerged from the dreaded door. My heart raced and my fingers traced the papers in my shaking hands for the sixth time. Taking three deep breaths, I followed her to the patient rooms; this was one of those "growing up" moments I had heard so much about lately. Reservations filled my head: Will she be nice like my pediatrician was, What is a physician assistant (PA), Am I ready for this? Jessica entered the room; her immediate demeanor put my doubts to ease. She began to get to know who I was, what my interests were, and her enthusiasm alleviated my anxiety. Her kind laughter filled the air when I handed her my medical records, the pediatrician already faxed everything over. Every visit since, Jessica would explain each procedure thoroughly, answer any questions I had, and inquire on my schooling. When she went on vacation, I realized I preferred using a PA. The other physicians at the practice gave the impression of being rushed and clinically observant. They did not give the notion of being comfortable and enthusiastic the way Jessica and the other PAs did. Her encouragement and confidence made me realize I wanted to work in health care.

Over the next several years, my interest in becoming a physician assistant has only strengthened with each experience in medicine. During my sophomore year of college, I began an unpaid internship for various departments at Riverside Community Hospital in California; a total of 373 beds accommodate a population over 300,000. From feeding patients, assisting in live births, and taking vital signs, I worked under the shadow of various providers for over 1.5 years. The most satisfying experiences were those where I spent time listening and talking with patients who did not receive many visitors. Their smiles were not only self gratifying, but they gave me a better sense of what healthcare can provide.

Consequently, I was able to witness the approach of the health care "team". In the Emergency Department (ED), I had my first hands-on experience with PAs. Through invaluable observation, I examined their adaptability, interpersonal skills, and how inquisitive each was. In the same way, they showed approachable leadership and confidence while maintaining self-discipline. Although interning was gratifying and rewarding, it left something inside me to be desired.

During the spring of 2012, I experienced a very unfortunate rock climbing accident and fractured my left tibia in 2 places. A few hours of surgery and 5 titanium screws propelled me into the healing process. An ill-fated consequence was the inability to ambulate for 4 weeks. My ultimate decision was to withdrawal from the quarter. Immediately, the frustration of simple life tasks such as taking a shower, brushing your teeth, and the ability to sit up overcame me as my leg atrophied. This unique experience granted me a patient insight. Greetings from a neighbor would drastically change my outlook for that day; appointments were treated like visits to Disneyland. These events provided me a positive outlook during my situation which I have employed in everyday life. It is not only bottles or pills that provide good medicine, but also the character and compassion of the health provider.

After graduation, I accepted a position in emergency medicine as an EMT working alongside other technicians and later the Los Angeles Fire Department. This area of healthcare has taught me how to work under conditions of high stress, allowing me to think independently in a versatile environment. It also educates me on the importance of life and the benefits preventative care provides. Most of the emergency situations I come across are avoidable and have shown me the significance of promoting beneficial routines while discouraging the harmful. The human body is a graceful machine; being a PA will not only give me the ability to positively influence peoples' lives, but allow me to work in rural areas where disparities in healthcare can be seen due to socioeconomic factors.

My desire to become a PA has been deeply rooted throughout my life. I plan on utilizing this training to work with the public in underserved urban areas along with rural. I have witnessed firsthand the deficiencies of healthcare in the United States and how communities experience hardship when effective care is not available. By utilizing my communication, critical thinking, and interpersonal skills, I sincerely believe I now have the qualities it takes to become a responsible and caring PA. I look forward to serving these diverse environments with empathy and compassion through the Physician Assistant Program.

Commentary Essay 42

You have an excellent start to your essay. The writing is descriptive and the essay flows well.

The main issue is that it's a little too focused on your personal experiences with illness and injury. Admissions Directors and faculty I interviewed want to hear less about that and more about your current work. That being said, you gained significant insight from your experiences and they should be included, just on an abbreviated scale. Then you'll have more room to focus on your current work. Pick a case or two that demonstrate the skills you've developed.

I'd delete the last sentence about your intern work. It undermines the value of that experience and is awkward the way it's written.

There are a few other awkward phrases and minor grammar errors. One way to catch those is to read the essay aloud. If your computer can do that for you, it's really helpful.

Essay 43

October 3, 2013. That was the day my dad told me that my grandfather had fallen after suffering a brain aneurysm at his farm in Ellsworth. My grandmother wasn't home at the time. They had lived on their farm in Ellsworth, KS for over 25 years. It's a town with a population of about 3000 people, spread across a large area of land and multiple family farms. That being said, by the time the ambulance reached the house from the town's local hospital, several more vessels in my grandfather's brain had weakened. When he arrived at ***************, my dad informed me that although they couldn't do much to fix the aneurysm, a family practice PA was able to stabilize my grandpa before airlifting him to ********** in Wichita. The next day, I had traveled to Wichita myself to find that my grandpa had since suffered multiple strokes and that the bleeding had now occupied nearly fifty percent of his brain. It was at that point that my family had made the decision to take my grandpa off life support. It had hit me like a ton of bricks. I had experienced death before; when I was little, but this was the first time I had truly seen it in person. It was the first time I had witnessed firsthand everything it took to keep a human life alive and well. The pain I was feeling was gut wrenching. After confirming his death, the nurse asked if we wanted to meet the medical staff that was in charge of my grandpa's care. I was shocked to learn that throughout that course of his stay, 2 different physicians and multiple physician assistants, of many different specialties, were responsible for making decisions regarding his care. It was at this point that I realized the compassion and versatility of the physician assistant profession. I had been interested in the PA program since high school, but it wasn't until this moment that I knew for certain that a PA is exactly the type of healthcare provider I wanted to be as it would give me the opportunity to serve those in my community that need help, without having to specialize in a particular field.

This passion to serve others has grown over the last several years as I have been given endless opportunities as student at Kansas State University. Perhaps the biggest blessing was obtaining a job as a CNA at the ***********. Despite being my first job in the healthcare system, I have learned and continue to learn knowledge regarding patient care and unique skills that are nearly impossible to obtain anywhere else. This job has allowed me to work with healthcare providers including multiple physician assistants in providing direct patient care, all while being a fulltime student. Never did I imagine that I would be able to order an MRI or CT for a patient and then be able to actually understand what the results meant. Never did I imagine that I would be able to take out sutures from a postoperative amputation one minute then apply a cast or splint to a little girl who broke her arm falling off of a swing the next minute.

Not only has this job taught me a wide array of skills that better allow me to serve in the healthcare field, but it has also allowed me to care for a variety of people, from multiple backgrounds. I was only working at the clinic for about a month when I had an experience with a patient that I will never forget. The receptionist came to the back, frustrated, because there was a Spanish speaking patient that needed help completing a health history form. She asked if there was anything we could do to help, thinking she would have to turn her away because no one knew how to help her or her son. No one was able to offer a solution. That was until I asked if I could see the chart. I had taken Spanish classes throughout high school and college, so I thought I could offer some assistance. I called the woman back to the room, and was able to help her complete the health history form. The woman appeared so thankful. Seeing the smile on her face when she realized that someone actually understood her gave me a sense of confidence. I then proceeded to ask her questions and obtain an intake about what her problem was. By that time, I was able to brief the physician on the problem and even translate the plan of care to the patient and her son. Although this process took a while as I struggled to correctly translate, I could tell the patient was very grateful for my effort. Before leaving she gave me a hug and said, "Gracias por tratarme como todos los otros". She wanted to thank me for treating her like everybody else.

This moment also confirmed for me that I belonged in a field that allows me to work closely with people. That is why I love the physician assistant job so much. I will be able to use my compassion and knowledge in multiple specialties to serve those like my grandpa, who need the most help.

Commentary Essay 43

You have a good start to your essay. The story about your grandfather is compelling — you have my condolences. However, you spent too much time talking about it. I would delete everything from the second sentence to "A family practice PA was able to stabilize him . . ."

Then I would skip the rest of the events until sadly, he passed away and the nurse asked if you wanted to meet the medical team. Then you can move to the sentence that starts, "I was shocked to learn . . ."

You've obtained a lot of good experience, and you're smart to write about it in your essay. Use the words you spent on your grandfather's story to write more about those experiences. Also, you mention briefly what you like about the PA profession, but you could definitely expand on that. Not having to specialize like MDs isn't the best of reasons for choosing the PA profession. CNAs, RNs and MDs all work closely with people, too. What's different about being a PA from your standpoint?

I like the story about the Spanish speaking patient. What she said is wonderful and should be included.

There are a couple of awkward sentences. For example, "This job has allowed me to work with healthcare providers including multiple physician assistants in providing direct patient care, all while being a full-time student."

Read each word in your essay and see if it's really necessary. Less if often more!

Essay 44

"Julie Wert 3 North" is the phrase I always remember hearing my mom say as she answered her work phone. At the time, my mom was working as charge nurse at Bayonet Point Hospital on the med surge unit. As a child what I loved about going to the hospital besides the graham crackers and juice boxes was seeing my mom work extremely hard for her patients but also for her staff. Reminiscing on our simple 15 minute hospital visits to see my mom really shows me where my love for medicine culminated from and where I originally began my journey into the medical field.

Since I have always had a love for medicine I began my journey by taking science courses at the community college while in high school. Once I had taken as many science courses that the community college could offer I transferred over to the University of South Florida (USF) to obtain a bachelor's degree in health sciences. Academically I am a dedicated and hardworking student. I take pride in my work ethic and continuously strive to always improve my range of knowledge. I truly believe that as a student and pre-physician assistant I am forever a lifelong learner which only invigorates me and challenges me to work that much harder every day.

Because I have been shadowing the diverse medical practices from primary care to plastic surgery I have been able to connect information I have learned from one field and apply it to a deeper understanding within another field. For example one patient whom was a 73 year old female was being prepped for surgery in the O.R. She was having her third squamous cell carcinoma removed from her right leg with a skin graft of her right inguinal region by Dr. Roach; the plastic surgeon who I shadow.

During the skin graft portion of the surgery I noticed that Dr. Roach had made a small nick in the epidermis of the skin graft before he sutured it onto the cancer free site. Postoperative before Dr.Roach begins his dictation of the surgery I asked him why he made the small hole in the skin graft and why he did not perform any cross hatching on the skin graft which I had seen done before by Sarah Yoho PA-C; the dermatology PA I shadow. He explained the reason a hole was made into the skin graft and when the technique of cross hatching is necessary. This particular example highlights how my knowledge learned through shadowing continues to build upon itself and allows me to see how delicately connected each field of medicine is to one another.

Now that I have talked about my academic integrity as well as passion for shadowing I need to discuss the part of the medical field which rarely gets addressed; stress management. I fully understand the high intensity and dedication PA school demands as I have spent the last two years preparing myself. Being a commuter to college as well as living between my brother's condo, my sister's apartment and my house with my mom I have obtained a strong regiment for time management and multitasking. On average my week consist of working morning shifts at Florida hospital of Tampa, shadowing, then heading off to my USF classes. I am able to handle the pressure of PA school because of my strong faith in Christ which grounds me and my family who stands firmly behind me in my journey to become a practicing PA.

All in all becoming a PA to me is more than diagnosing and helping others; becoming a PA is a lifelong path that God has lead me to. Being a PA means you are a part of a new family whose goals are to improve the medical care our patients receive and to make our patients feel like they are part of our family as well. I know my abilities and I know the work I am willing to put forth to have my name read Stephanie Wert PAC.

Commentary Essay 44

Your essay has some good information, but it's hard to appreciate the content because the essay is literally hard to read. The sentences are long and completely devoid of commas. Your reader is trying to figure out what you're trying to write instead of appreciating what you say. Also, it lacks any explanation about why you want to be a PA, which is supposed to be the whole point of the essay. Instead of writing about Dr. Roach, write about a PA shadowing experience. Show what the PA did and tell why that appeals to you.

The paragraph about stress management assumes that people don't talk about the topic much. Actually, it's a very common topic in these essays. Take a different approach to starting that paragraph, especially the opening words: "Now that I have talked about my academic integrity as well as passion for shadowing . . ." They're very informal for this type of an essay.

Your conclusion right now is weak. Once you've written about why you want to be a PA, you'll have more information to draw from to write a strong conclusion.

Essay 45

I was first introduced to the physician assistant profession in the waiting room of Banner Cordon Hospital when I was only thirteen. My great grandmother, Kathryn, was currently being seen after she was found in her home struggling to move due to an immense pain in her abdomen. As I sat with my family, I experienced emotions that I never had to feel before, the fear of losing someone. As I sat without her in that waiting room, I never felt more alone. My great grandmother had been someone that was always present in my life. The physician assistant that was in charge of her care came into the waiting room. She walked over and introduced herself (I will call her Emily), pulled up a chair, looked at us with a tone of sorrow in her voice and said, "I'm sorry, but it looks like Kathryn has something we call liver cirrhosis, and it is highly progressed." She explained to us what causes this condition and what we were to expect in the coming days. She didn't act rushed and she made us feel like an important part of my great grandmother's case. Following that day, she was moved into hospice, as she was only given a couple of weeks. After her body began to further succumb to her condition, we decided it would be best to move her to her home so she could be comfortable in her final days. When relaying our decision to Emily, she gave us her personal number and told us to call the minute anything were to change. Two days later, after moving my great grandmother back home, she stopped breathing. We then called Emily, after calling EMS, and rushed her to the ER. Emily met us at ambulance bay and helped rush her to a bed. An hour of grueling waiting passed by, and Emily came out to tell us that my great grandmother had passed. Nearly ten years later since her passing, I look back and realize that Emily's dedication to her patients and caring demeanor are traits that first drew me to the fulfilling profession of a physician assistant.

During my time at Arizona State University, while working towards my BS in biological sciences, I took a clinical research position in the behavioral sciences department. In this position, I was able to spend working with overweight students to help develop a plan for obesity prevention. One of my goals was to use nutrition and exercise with many other factors like sleep, to aide these students in obtaining and living healthier lives. The study was quite successful with many of the students losing more than 20 pounds following the 6 weeks of the study. I was first drawn to this position, because the study didn't turn anyone away. As long as a patient meets the inclusion criteria for the study, they were allowed to enroll and begin to lead healthier lives. My students helped me realize what struggles many people go through to become better and made me yearn to continue helping others to strive towards a better life. By providing an additional source of care, PAs can help to reduce the amount of people that are unable to get help for their conditions. I strive to become part of this initiative and work as part of a team that provides exceptional and personalized care.

I started working in the medical field during my senior year of college. I began working as an optometrist technician in a small practice. Nevertheless, I have learned quickly and was fascinated with the responsibility of "pretesting" patients for the optometrist, such as measuring their visual fields and their intraocular pressures. I am currently still apart of this practice and have learned a lot about the medical field, however this was only a stepping stone to my sole passion. Towards the end of my senior year, I decided to start working as an Emergency Room medical scribe to gain as much exposure to the professions of PAs, MDs, Dos, and NPs. As a medical scribe, I gained additional patient care experience and an increased burn of passion to get into the medical field. Emergency medicine opened my eyes to the diversity of each situation, between each patient's unique history and the steps taking for each and every treatment. Each patient I had the privilege of meeting with had distinct motivations to become better, and through varying levels of support each provider I worked with made it their goal to treat each patient to the highest of standards. Just as illness affects a patient's life, each patient's unique life story greatly influences his or her ability to overcome illness, and in the emergency room time also becomes a factor. Through my scribing experiences, I learned that the PAs I have worked alongside often have the time to get to know patients on the level that is necessary to take all of these factors into consideration even in the emergency room. This is not because Pas are less busy, or have more compassion than their counterparts. Instead, the role of a PA often includes discussing treatment and educating the patient on what the next steps are in their healing process, seeing them as a person, not just a diagnosis. My motivation to become a PA has only enhanced itself by observing medical professionals. However, the PA profession complements my goal to become a healthcare provider who weighs all factors when assisting patients and ensuring that their families are included during all sections of their treatment.

I have always dreamed of having a career that is fulfilling and significant. My decision to pursue the PA profession is built upon a solid foundation of working alongside different healthcare professionals along with my college work. A career as a PA will allow me to use the strengths of my being to further make a difference in people's lives and strive to give people a better, healthier, longer lasting life.

Commentary Essay 45

The key to the success of your essay will be concision — right now it is well over the CASPA limit. A great place to start is your first paragraph. I'd edit it to this (with a caveat — I added some words of my own):

"I was first introduced to the physician assistant profession in the waiting room of Banner Cordon Hospital when I was only thirteen. My adored great grandmother, Kathryn, was being seen after she experienced severe abdominal pain. As I sat without her in that waiting room, I never felt more alone. The physician assistant who was in charge of her care walked into the room, introduced herself (I will call her Emily), pulled up a chair, and with a tone of sorrow said, "I'm sorry, but Kathryn has liver cirrhosis, and it is highly progressed." She explained the cause and what we could expect in the coming days. She did not act rushed and she made us feel like an important part of my great grandmother's case. Emily gave us her personal number and told us to call if we needed her. Nearly ten years later, I can look back and realize that Emily's dedication to her patients and caring demeanor are traits that first drew me to the fulfilling profession of physician assistant."

With the edits you save almost 1000 characters and spaces. That gives you room to write the need transition to the second paragraph, which by the way has problems. While most of the essay is great, the second paragraph is a weak point because conclusion is unrelated to its content. You'll need to work on that. Otherwise, just go through the essay and scrutinize every word to see if it's necessary. With concision (and transitions), you'll have a great essay.

Essay 46

During my senior year of high school I had an unexpected visit to the doctor. While preparing for my last season of wrestling, my peroneal tendons began to slide over my lateral malleolus. It was to the point where it became painful enough to seek treatment. I intended to see an orthopedic physician, but instead I was seen by the physician assistant (PA).

As the nurse called my name, a plethora of emotions flooded my mind. I was anxious to ascertain what was wrong, relieved to understand the source of my pain, but the feeling that took over the most was fear. I was worried that I would not be able to compete in a sport that I was not only passionate about, but one that has helped shape who I am today, wrestling. I cannot remember a time when wrestling wasn't an integral part of my life. It not only taught me leadership, determination, and discipline, it was also an adjunct to the relationship with my father.

As I tried to make sense of all the thoughts in my mind the PA walked in. He could tell by the look on my face that I was upset, and immediately he sat down and asked me to explain what happened, how I was feeling, and what I wanted to do about it. It was evident that he cared about what I wanted, and he was understanding about my feelings towards wrestling. He discussed the treatment options, and together we made the decision that I would treat my ankle conservatively until wrestling season was over. He made me feel at ease, and for the first time I felt important at a doctor's office. The office was busy and full of patients, but the PA made sure to take the extra time to reassure me that everything was going to be okay. Every time I came in for a follow up appointment I received the exact same care as the initial consult. It exemplified how a PA works autonomously treating patients, and is able to form personal and trusting relationships with each one.

This experience solidified my desire to pursue a profession in medicine. I have always been interested in the sciences. My goals and aspirations led me to Ithaca College where I majored in exercise science with an emphasis in medical sciences. My major allowed me to fulfill my passion for sports and fitness, while also providing essential qualities and attributes required for the medical field. Since I continued to wrestle in college, shadowing a PA during the summer was the most convenient for me. As I was shadowing, I was able to better understand the profession, along with the skills and qualities needed to become a successful PA. While each PA has their own unique experiences, all of them seem to share similar goals in the healthcare profession; providing quality medical care and having the ability to treat and diagnose patients.

After graduating college I began taking an EMT class while volunteering at the community rescue squad. This expanded my health care knowledge and patient care experience, while also allowing me to help out my community. While at the rescue squad, I concurrently worked as a Patient Care Assistant in the emergency department at a hospital. Between both jobs I was exposed to high stress situations that required important decision making. As an EMT, the patients receiving care are in their most vulnerable state physically and emotionally. I've learned how to stay calm in chaotic situations, while assuring the patient they could trust and depend on me. Becoming an EMT not only provided me with the ability to treat those needing medical attention, but more importantly how to effectively handle and communicate with patients in a timely manner.

Currently I am working as a Telemetry Technician in a long term acute care unit. After taking an EKG class I now am responsible for determining EKG rhythms and to notify the RN's of any waveform alterations or abnormalities. Understanding what different waves and segments mean and how they correspond to the heart is so awesome! I love when the Cardiologists come up to talk to me because I try to pick their brains as much as I can with questions.

Both my education and experiences in the healthcare field have helped me develop skills and qualities that are expected of a PA. I have learned how to communicate with patients, help them cope with negative situations, and how to care about each patient individually and in a professional manner. My work experience has also helped me learn organizational skills and time management. I believe my work experience has been a monumental stepping stone on my journey to become a PA.

In becoming a PA, I will become a crucial member of a team of healthcare professionals. Through my experiences I have learned the importance of teamwork, and am fully committed to becoming a PA. In wrestling, when given a challenge I overcame it through devotion and desire. I plan on facing the rigor of the PA curriculum with the same attitude and I will dedicate myself to becoming the best possible Physician Assistant.

Commentary Essay 46

You've done a really good job on your essay. Still, I have a few suggestions.

First, shorten the second two paragraphs into one concise paragraph. Yes, your injury was the catalyst for your interest in medicine and your introduction to the PA profession, but Admissions Directors want to hear more about your adult experiences than your youthful, personal experiences.

Then use the extra space to write about experiences you've had while working. You're good at setting the scene. Do it for a situation you experienced as an EMT or while shadowing to illustrate some of the points you make about your skills.

Omit the word "awesome" and the exclamation point. Use a more professional word. Also, I don't think you need the sentence about picking the cardiologist's brains. It really doesn't add anything, and seems less polished than the rest of the essay.

Consider separating the final paragraph into two, perhaps starting with "In becoming a PA . . ." That way it seems more like a conclusion to your essay.

Essay 47

I know that my essay is way too long. I appreciate any help in what you think can be cut out or condensed. Please rip it apart and provide feedback. I'm not great with grammar but my brother in-law is a English professor, he's going to help me there.

When people ask me, "What kind of medical experience do you have?" I always answer with the same reply, "I did a chest tube on the side of a mountain in Afghanistan."

At the terminal end of high school, I was clueless to where I would fit in the world – life at the time was a cacophony of choices. As much as I didn't know, I knew that I was not mature enough for college. Like my father, grandpa and great grandpa, I enlisted in the US Navy. I've always known that I wanted to do health care; so becoming a combat medic (Corpsman) assigned to infantry Marines seemed natural. After 3 years, I was the senior medical provider for India Company and the senior of 10 other enlisted medics. It wasn't until my deployment to Afghanistan where I realized what I was born to do.

I was quietly resting in my cave after a long patrol when suddenly, an explosion and echoing cracks of machine gun fire broke the silence of the twilight. Grabbing my file, I ran outside and rallied up with my Marines to hunt the insurgents who attack us. Abruptly after moving only a hundred feet from our base, every ounce of light and consciousness left me. I immediately came around in an unfocused haze accented by a deafening high pitch tone. I knew someone had just stepped on an explosive booby-trap.

Exhausted, bent over and on my knees, I griped the warm dirt. I registered the hysteria of a grown man and while still taking fire from the enemy, I stood up and made my way to the Marine. My friend, *******, had both his legs traumatically removed. He was blinded by pain he was screaming in intense hysterical pain. As I assessed and treated his injuries, the screaming stopped. He was no longer grabbing and clawing at me. ****** let out a few agonal breaths and closed his eyes forever. I saved multiple trauma victims in Afghanistan, but it's the ones I failed that will stay with me. His death is the catalyst of my motivation, my motivation to be better in every way and to have no regrets because I didn't accomplish my dreams.

Under these conditions is when you're the most honest with yourself. I spent a lot of time with physician assistants (PA) in the clinic at my previous duty station. The PAs were always the providers that were in there with the patient. Periodically they consulted with the physicians but on the whole, they were the ones doing the real care. I observed this again with rotations to other hospitals and again during my shadowing, I knew that's the kind of provider I want to be, the upper echelon of care that still routinely kept hands on the patient every day. Following discussions with physicians, PAs, family and friends, I knew that my time in the service was over. I wanted to become a PA, it became my dream and that is what I was going to do.

When I initially started college I thought I knew I was ready for school, I had been though war – twice. I learned though, higher education is a different type of toil. I definitely found myself stumbling but after my first year, I finally got my feet underneath me. By facing my failures, I improved myself. I found out that if I studied with others, I enjoyed the challenge of the hard classes; we enjoyed the teamwork of pushing each other hard. Nothing felt better than the satisfaction of a high grade after days, weeks and months of no reprieve. Even though I initially did not receive the best marks, I finally figured out what fueled me – the pride of hard work.

After three of my four grandparents were diagnosed with Alzheimer's Disease, I became an activist. Whether fate or coincidence, Dr. **** invited me to join his research group were they were investigating novel AD treatments. Any spare time I had, I dedicated to being an active participant in the solution of AD. I developed with graduate students, an idea that lead to a research grant that changed the direction of the entire research group and led to a publication.

Through my observations and experiences with PAs, it obvious that they're leaders within their environment. Although I had ample experience as a leader throughout the military, I wanted leadership experience in academia. To that end, I volunteered to be a chemistry supplemental instructor where I lead tutoring sessions of 30 or more students. After being asked to return in subsequent semesters because of my ethics, knowledge and communication skills. I also became a teaching assistant for the anatomy and physiology course where I equally excelled. In both instances, my leadership and communication resulted in higher grades for the students.

I didn't choose nursing because I know that I have the ability to be that higher echelon of medical care. I've proven that I have the capacity to work in collaboration with physicians and to be the conduit of direct contact with patients and to preform interventions. I love the fact that PAs are nicknamed, " the jack of all trades" because they receive training in all specialties. Simply, the ability to operate right at the level of a physician but maintain a high level of patient contact is why I chose to be PA. I love the idea of empowering doctors to focus on their strengths by shouldering some of their burden. To me, a physician's assistant serves not only their patients, but also their doctor as well. I want my career to be focused on the patient and the intimate trust between the physician and health care team in order to deliver excellent healthcare to patients. I do not want to focus on insurance, impersonal care and the business of medicine.

Once I complete PA school and begin my life's career, one thing I am desperate to do is mentor. I finished high school with a 1.2 GPA, rose though the ranks of the Navy, defeated my Afghanistan induced PTSD, immersed myself in undergraduate research and teaching, graduated from college with a BS in biological science and finally, earned the title of a PA. I want to guide others the way I was by so many, I want to show others that if you have the courage to be successful, you can become or do anything. Becoming a PA is not the end for me; it's the next step in creating the change in the world I want to see – people caring for people.

Commentary Essay 47

You've done such amazing things and survived horrendous experiences and challenges. You have much to write about, and that makes it hard to make many specific suggestions in a forum like this.

One of the first things you might want to do is cut back on some of the description of your friend's dying moments. His death was horrific, and you've written about it in a way that made me feel like I was there for every agonizing moment. But less might be more in the context of the essay.

If necessary for space, you could leave out the Alzheimer's research project information. It's not as important as the other things you've done.

It's great that you decided to help with the teaching. It shows your leadership skills and ability to communicate, two important traits for PAs. The paragraph has repetition, though, so take a look and see where you've made the same point more than once and cut those sentences/phrases.

The paragraph that begins "I didn't choose nursing . . ." is long. You could make your point in a couple of sentences. Also, I'm not sure it benefits you to say that PAs operate at the level of the doctor. You could leave that out.

Your final paragraph could be revised. Instead of focusing on mentoring people after you've become a PA, focus on your accomplishments and how that will help you be a PA. I love the last sentence, though. It's wonderful.

I won't make any grammar comments since you have an English professor to do that.

My heartfelt thanks go to you for all you've done.

Essay 48

Surrounded by the sizzle of cooking meat, 'Carol' and I worked together to make the night's meal. She hosts a dinner for friends every week, and I like to help out beforehand when I have the chance. "Mind if we switch jobs," I asked, "I can't seem to slice this cheese evenly, and I would much rather flip those burgers." While I am certainly not the best cheese slicer around, this wasn't my real motivation for asking. My friend was beginning to look tired, and I wanted to give her the break she seemed to need without her having to ask for help. Carol is proud, and she has multiple sclerosis.

Empathy is a hard thing. We feel pain that is not ours, and wonder how and why the world became so cruel. Science, for me, has always provided the answer to those questions. Science helps me to see the larger context within which both joy and suffering are happening, and to distance myself from the pain that often comes with empathy. Science is the answer to the how and the why, and within that answer I thought to find serenity.

Working as a biological field technician, I was initially content collecting samples and observing nature. Rarely seeing another person, I was at first dazzled by how the 'open space' and 'empty air' were completely filled with so many lives, but it didn't take long for me to understand that there was something missing. I couldn't find the meaning in what I was doing. What difference was I making? It began to occur to me that the questions I had been asking were the wrong ones, and that I had therefore gotten the wrong answer. Science could provide distance from pain, but distance from sad and painful things doesn't make them better. The real question I needed to answer wasn't how or why the world is cruel, but rather, 'what can we, and I in particular, do to have a positive impact?'

As is my tradition, I looked for a solution using a combination of research and process of elimination. I love biology, and knew that I wanted to work within that field, but my technician job and time involved in student government had shown me that making connections with people is where I find meaning. This almost certainly means healthcare if you actually want a job, but that is a broad category. It was while working as a residence assistant that I learned that I am happiest when working under a mentor, and that a high level of autonomy is important to me. With that knowledge I had my answer, physician assistant, and I began to work toward my goal. ASIDE: I know this needs work . . . suggestions?

Since I go to school in one of the poorest counties in Iowa, I knew that I wasn't likely to get a part time job in health care, and I wouldn't want to take a paying job from someone who needed it anyway. Therefore, I decided to volunteer instead, and I knew where there was the most need. Very few people are comfortable talking to and being with a hospice patient, but I am glad that I chose to be a hospice volunteer. There are times when the silence seems heavy, but there is also something special about being with a person who is near the end of their life.

Empathy is still hard, and harder still when there is nothing you can do to make things better. What are you supposed to do when you can't help someone? What do you say to or do for a person who is terminally ill? Carol herself gave me the answer. "All you can say is that you're sorry, and all you can do is be with them.

Commentary Essay 48

Your empathy comes through in spades. Your patients will be lucky. But for your essay, I think you need more. Rather than spending so much time in your second two paragraphs pondering, talk about your hospice experiences and any others you may have had (if you shadowed a PA, for example), and what you've gained from them. Hospice volunteers do so much. I know you have things to write about.

I recommend that you leave this out: "Since I go to school in one of the poorest counties in Iowa, I knew that I wasn't likely to get a part time job in health care, and I wouldn't want to take a paying job from someone who needed it anyway." There's a better way to lead in to your decision to volunteer.

Your fourth paragraph doesn't do what you hope it will. It's quite a leap from RA/bio field technician to PA and we're missing the connection. How did you learn about the profession? Did you have contact with PAs? How did you start to work toward that goal? You'll have to explain it.

The biggest issue I see in your essay is that your readers won't know anything about you except that you have empathy and are a thinking person. Those are great qualities, but you have to be more specific about why being a PA is the right profession for you, and why you'd be a good candidate for PA school. Bring your essay down to earth a bit, and you'll be in good stead.

Essay 49

During my semester abroad, my teacher of Peruvian Culture and Society and I went to interview Martha in a small Quechua village in the Andes. In these villages, there were no public resources such as schools or hospitals within walking distance, which in effect, created a lack of education. Many of the older community members, including Martha, spoke neither Spanish nor English but only their native language, Quechua. As we were interviewing her and having tea, she casually took out a condom. We were curious, but waited to see what she was doing with it.

She opened the wrapper, unraveled it, and dipped it in her tea as she would a tea bag. Stunned, my teacher had to ask why she was doing this. She explained that these "voluntarios" came to the village and gave them condoms and told them that they protected against diseases. Her statement has remained close to my heart and has been one of the many sources driving my passion of helping those who are uneducated.

This passion stemmed from my upbringing. Growing up with Chippewa Cree roots, I have witnessed the lack of desire to be educated or helped and the importance of traditional beliefs. This lack of knowledge, in turn, led to negligence and malnutrition. With a childhood in a young, single mother household, I have also seen how easy it is to disregard the importance of health and knowledge. A struggling mother does not always worry about "clean eating" when holding a minimum wage job.

For many people, this cycle of poverty, addiction, and ignorance seems to be a never-ending ordeal from generation to the next. However, I broke the cycle after I moved out of that environment when I was 15. There is no denying that it was a challenging time, but more importantly, it was a time for growth. I grew immensely through the next few years through the discovery of the power of education. After the growth away from my previous environment, I saw it in a different light and realized the unhealthiness that came along with poverty. I decided that with my love of science and passion for education, I was going to help communities like mine through the field of medicine.

During my first year of college, I was still determined to pursue health care, but I was not quite sure what branch to leap for. I had not even heard of the position of Physician Assistant until my sister explained the career to me. I went to visit a couple of

Physician Assistants in my hometown and after seeing how one of them took the time to explain exactly why the acidity in cranberry juice helps prevent infection, I know that this was going to be my profession. Further research on Physician Assistants affirmed my certainty because of the continuing learning while practicing medicine. I knew this would be the best route not only in helping people, but in showing them how powerful they can be with knowledge.

In order to gain some experience in health care, I began working as a Nurse's Aide at an assisted living home for residents with Alzheimer's disease and dementia. The work can be very challenging and there have been many times that being punched and kicked almost became too much. But every now and then, while helping a resident into bed or bringing them a snack, they look at me and say, "Thank you for doing everything that you do." This simple appreciation reminds me that under their terrible disease, they are just people who need a little help and I am thankful that I get to work with a team that provides the quality of help that they deserve. The challenge of this job has been an enormous growing experience and taught me communication skills on a different level along with the importance of teamwork. Most importantly, the residents have taught me empathy, compassion, and solidified my certainty of caring for people who do not always know how to care for themselves.

Throughout college, preparing for a physician assistant has also been a time of growth. With a major of Hispanic Studies, I have had to juggle knowledge on two different sides of the spectrum. The struggle of using both extremes of my brain has taught me to be proactive and organize my time effectively. Along with science, I have also learned a completely different culture through school and studying and volunteering in South America. Although challenging at many times, studying science and Hispanic Studies has made me more well-rounded and has broadened my passion.

Throughout my life, I have realized the importance of education in the health field. Living and experiencing the effects of ignorance has made me determined to help those who are still experiencing them discover aspects of their health that they may not be aware of. I know that I will do this through the Physician Assistant profession whether it be in South America or my own backyard.

Commentary Essay 49

Excellent job on your essay. You've made important points about key components of the PA profession — education, compassion, organization, working in stressful situations, communication. Now you need to tie them to your goal of becoming a PA.

The fourth paragraph is the weakest section. There are a dozen ways to educate people as a health professional. You will need to elaborate on why you chose the PA route as opposed to another. Visiting "a couple" of PAs is vague, and telling how one of them explained the effects of cranberry juice on infections isn't strong. Have you shadowed PAs? What did your research reveal? Do you interact with PAs in your job? Talk about some of those things. What else about being a PA appeals to you? There's a lot more to the job than educating people.

Your conclusion, too, focuses solely on the importance of education in the health field. It would be helpful to expand on that to include more aspects of the PA profession that are important to you.

You can shorten the essay a bit. Reread it carefully and see where you make the same point more than once. This sentence, for example, merely recaps what you've said throughout the essay: "Along with science, I have also learned a completely different culture through school and studying and volunteering in South America."

Remember, your readers are seeing 1,000-2,000 essays each admissions season. You want to make your essay as concise as possible.

Essay 50

"What is moyamoya?" I asked my charge nurse as I reviewed the diagnosis for Ms. P, a new patient. After she explained how it affects a patient's cerebrovascular system, I headed to Ms. P's room saying moyamoya under my breath a few more times, considering its foreign tone. Little did I know, caring for Ms. P would greatly teach and test me as a CNA and care provider over the next several months. Due to her condition, she was frequently disoriented and exhibited extreme emotional swings, going from intensely grateful towards me in one moment to dishearteningly condescending the next, even accusing me of wanting her to feel pain during personal cares. While some coworkers asked to trade patients so they would not have to care for her, I found myself more than willing to do so to ensure she would be cared for by someone who wanted to be there.

It was by no means easy, as her emotional swings could be mentally draining, but her moments of clarity, like when she was truly thankful I was able to feed her or able to crack a joke about politics, made it all worth it. One morning I walked into her room in a tired, irritable mood. Ms. P was already awake, and said, "Thank goodness you're here I had a terrible night." Her words snapped me back into my usual positive and engaging self. That moment was a culmination of my months of diligent care. It solidified how paramount it is to always provide patients with a consistent and empathetic attitude, as interactions with them can be what make or break their day and bring them joy or sorrow. Moments like this are what drive me to become a PA.

It takes many such moments to truly be comfortable with a career decision, and not long ago I was frequently thinking "What am I going to do with my life?" The question has been a fear lingering in my mind all throughout college. Thankfully fears often drive results. My journey to the answer has included exploring multiple careers, including PT, OT, public health, and more before finding the PA profession. I have volunteered in a PT clinic, spent over a year serving working towards occupational and speech therapy goals with a young boy who has autism, among others. While understanding those fields' principles and merits will be useful in my future, they never truly captivated me. Exploring and analyzing becoming a PA has steadily eradicated that fear. During my second shadowing experience, a family practice PA I have been learning from validated my feelings that each patient interaction is a puzzle requiring critical thinking. I have been in awe at times, watching him deftly integrate patient history, body language, complaints, and manifestations to finish the puzzle by recommending lifestyle change, prescribing medicine, ordering imaging, etc. His ability to provide so much in a condensed period of time is remarkable. Post-visit discussions of what key points or techniques led him to his answer have made me eager to one day wear those shoes. Like with Ms. P, the hours I have shadowed PAs have been more of those moments pushing me towards becoming a PA.

My favorite aspect about working on a sub-acute rehab and nursing unit has been caring for a wide variety of patients, as some may be in for a few days of IV antibiotics, while others may have serious complications requiring demanding therapy such as Ms. P's case. With this patient pool, the variety of healthcare professionals I interact with on a daily basis is also broad. I've developed a strong appreciation of how important teamwork and collaboration are to the healing process. Knowing that if I fail to be there when a patient needs me to help get ready for therapy could set his whole day back drives me to be efficient and detail oriented. I double check my patient therapy schedules each shift to ensure I do my part to maintain their personal schedule. Watching physicians and PAs routinely look to nurses for explanation of their patient's normal behavior is inspiring. Advancing to become a PA would allow me to use my knowledge and problem solving skills to be a more effective and valuable part of the team.

The objectives that require the most perseverance to reach in life often require a mindset formed and solidified through personal reflection to achieve them. When my mother asked why I wanted to be a PA when I was in the early stages of exploring it, I did not have an answer I was comfortable with. Months after learning more about myself and the profession, I was able to confidently explain to her. I believe in my heart and mind that there is no worthier pursuit than improving other people's time on earth, as time is the only resource we all have. While many routes can be taken to achieve that, I've found my interpersonal communication skills, ability to empathize with others, and understand science and medicine have lead me to moments that have driven me to become a PA.

Commentary Essay 50

I really love the opening line. It's priceless. To tie it into Ms. P, you could add to this sentence as I've suggested: "Little did I know, caring for Ms. P would greatly teach and test me as a CNA and care provider, and not just because of her diagnosis.

Overall you have done a great job in the essay. The transitions are good for the most part. You need one for the paragraph that starts with "My favorite aspect about working on a sub-acute rehab . . ."

You could do without this somewhat convoluted and general statement: "The objectives that require the most perseverance to reach in life often require a mindset formed and solidified through personal reflection to achieve them." Keep things personal to you, and skip the philosophy.

Other than that, and using "etc." (never use it — be specific) and contractions (they're disfavored in academic essays), you've got an excellent essay.

Essay 51

I was in the passenger seat giving directions to my house in the rural part of town.   Just a half mile away from home, I realized we were going too fast, and soon our car was going straight toward an eight-foot ditch. I braced myself as a sharp pain shot through my lower back, and I lost control of my left arm. An ambulance ride later, I was at the hospital diagnosed with a fractured humerus, ribs, and a lacerated liver. I was in absolute shock; these were my first broken bones as well as my first car accident.

While recovering from surgery and the emotional trauma, the treatment of the staff flowing in and out of my room remains a distinct memory. Among the staff was Christina, a physician assistant (PA). Christina actually sat with me and truly listened to my concerns and advised ways in which I was able to improve my experience on the otherwise mundane hospital bed. Also remarkable was that she spoke with me longer than most doctors did and explained more to me than nurses could. Christina was the most comforting and informative source during one of the most traumatic experiences of my life. The extra time taken by the PA incorporating teachable moments into her bedside manner made a lasting impression.

Five years later, I now work in the same hospital and operating room (OR) in which I received my surgery, and it is an everyday reminder that my recovery and productivity is a direct result of these medical professionals. Being integrated into this team has reinforced my decision to become a PA by teaching me how to be a better communicator, make quick decisions, and remain compassionate. As a current Arterial Monitor Technician, I have experienced numerous surgeries in most specialties, including level I trauma surgeries, and have learned how to carry out my duties while continuously collaborating with the rest of the team.

While the majority of my time with patients consists of them under general anesthesia, I cherish an instance in which an elderly patient had to be awake during her neurological surgery. As she was wheeled into the OR, she gripped a photo collage of her family. Being almost entirely an intraoperative employee, it is rare that I have the privilege of seeing into the true lives of our patients, and I wanted to know more. As her local anesthetic was being prepared, she was naming the smiling faces in her photos, and we assured her that she would see them all again. Once the operation was underway, there were times where she needed consolation. Because it was my responsibility to ensure that her arterial line in her radial artery was secure, I had easy access to her hand, and whenever she seemed to be in distress, I held her hand and her comforted expression touched me in a way that I had not experienced before.

I desire to play a bigger role in patients' treatment and not be confined exclusively to intraoperative care. Kara, a PA I shadow in vascular surgery, has the opportunity to not only assist surgeons in the OR, but also to consult patients before surgery and then follow up with postoperative care. Having the ability to be more responsible for a patient's overall care and health is my big motivation.

I would be very grateful for the opportunity to prove my enthusiasm through the PA program. The experiences I have had in the operating room and shadowing have elucidated some of the obstacles I expect to face, such has difficult decision making and continuous education, but I welcome them. I know I can overcome challenges with my drive and determination as I have proven in the past to both others and myself. I excelled during my undergraduate career and then again with efficiently learning new jobs and skills in positions that were once unfamiliar. As a PA, I would strive to educate patients about their health and work towards making a positive impact, no matter how small, to the field of medicine.

Commentary Essay 51

Great essay. I can tell you've done a lot of work to get to this point. You've covered the main points necessary and done it well.

The conclusion is a bit weak, especially the first sentence. Read it again and see if it really delivers the message you hope readers will take from the essay. I think you'll conclude that proving your enthusiasm is not a very good reason to become a PA. I recommend that you delete that sentence.

The last sentence is weak as well. It should be the one that ties up the entire essay. Delete the first sentence and rework the last sentence and you'll have a strong essay.

Essay 52

"Code trauma bed 8." "Code trauma bed 8." Code trauma bed 8."

The overhead speaker calmly alerted the emergency department (ED) staff towards a patient requiring immediate care. This was my first exposure to injury of any kind, serious or otherwise, and, believe it or not, was also my first day working as a scribe in the emergency room. As the physician and I walked towards bed 8, I remember feeling very anxious and simultaneously excited for the new experience.

After graduating college, I was unable to find work. With student loan payments about to roll in I felt desperate to find a job, any job. I was hired at Payless that summer and at Brighton Collectibles in the fall, both customer service positions.

I had an interest in medicine however, as I graduated college with an impressive accumulation of debt, the idea of pursuing any further education seemed overwhelming. When a friend of mine offered me a position as a scribe in the ED, I took it. At this time, I left my position at Payless and moved forward with one position in customer service at Brighton and working as a scribe in the emergency department.

The patient was young, my age, writhing in pain and screaming for her friends. Friends, who we later learned were all killed in a traffic accident. Standing at the end of her gurney, I watched as, the doctor, PA, nurses, emergency room technicians (EMTs) and a few fire personnel all huddled into the room. It was a well-rehearsed orchestra. The entire team working together with one purpose; to utilize their skills in helping the patient.

The doctor was calling out to me, telling me the patient's story and physical exam findings. "Superficial abrasion to the left lateral calf." "No seat belt sign." "Abdomen soft and nontender."

Listening to her screams I felt so helpless. To experience true fear and to put a face to those emotions in someone, who very well could be yourself, a friend or a relative, is truly an unforgettable experience. I felt an overwhelming desire to help, however I could. As it was my first day as a scribe, what could I do?

Working in the Emergency Department at Inland Valley was an invaluable and eye opening experience. As a scribe, I worked side by side with the physician and physician assistant. Together, we go directly to the patients bedside and I document their assessment of the patient; I help to write the chart. Working various shifts in a level 4 trauma center gave me exposure to various medical careers.

In order to increase my exposure to medicine I took a second scribing position in 2013 at Corona Regional Medical Center, a level 2 trauma hospital. The acuity of the patients was much different. In discussion with the medical providers I learned that, as the only hospital in the area, they after see a high volume of patients with a lower acuity.

Between the two site, I was able to see an incredible variety of medical cases. While working as a scribe in two different emergency rooms, I have also been working in a retail/customer service position. Working side by side with the PA, we together saw patients. At my site, the scribe goes to the bedside of every patient that the physician assistant sees and documents the encounter in the electronic medical record (EMR). I have learned how to document a medical encounter; the history of present illness (HPI) and how it should differ from the review of systems (ROS). The PAs I met are incredible and so supportive of our goals to enter medicine. We were allowed to watch lumbar punctures, laceration repairs, foreign body removals, cardioversions....everything. As long as you ask, you will be included.

Their encouragement inspired me to go back to school and complete the remainder of my prerequisites. Working in the ED definitely reminds you how fragile life can be. After witnessing that first trauma and with positive words of encouragement, I will also embark on a solo volunteer trip to Guatemala to teach children good hygiene behaviors.

Between working in retail for so many years, I definitely took away two very important lessons. The first, retail is not what I am passionate about. The second being that I have been put in so many positions, talking to so many different people that I have learned how to ask the right questions and how to communicate effectively. This translates well to the ED, when encountering a new patient, what questions do you ask? When the patient answers, are they really answering your question or did they go off topic? How do you reroute the conversation so that they understand what you are asking them? Communication is incredibly important and this skill will be incredibly helpful as a PA.

I aspire to become a Physician Assistant who genuinely cares for their patients. I believe one of the greatest resources PAs can provide is not only compassion but the ability to take the time and educate your patients. With more insured Americans and the influx of patients on every provider, more offices are looking to hire PAs. I will be one of those who is willing to take the time and communicate with my patient about their health; past, present and future.

Commentary Essay 52

I can tell you've spent a lot of time on your essay. I like the way you've tied your life/medical experience together.

A few suggestions: You only need one "Code trauma bed 8." In fact, it's more effective as a stand-alone sentence to open your essay. Otherwise, the repetition undermines the urgency.

The second paragraph is out of place, and I'm thinking your third paragraph isn't helpful. You've started with a very vivid story, and then completely switch subjects.

Saying you couldn't find any job and that a friend offered you a scribe job probably isn't a good idea. The lack of jobs may be true (as it has been for many college students due to the economy), but you want to stand out in a positive, not negative way. You don't want readers to wonder if something made you unemployable. You mention that you've worked retail while you worked as a scribe. That's enough. Then your paragraph about how working retail taught you important lessons works great.

There are a few grammar type errors. "Between the two site," should be "Between the two sites," and the sentence that begins "Between working in retail for so many years," is awkward. Plus, you don't want to start two sentences in a short essay with "Between."

Watch your verbs so you don't use past and present tense in the same sentence. Don't use ellipses (which if anything would be three, not four), use an em dash instead —.

Essay 53

When getting advice for writing a personal statement for Physician Assistant school I was told first and foremost not to say that I have "always known" that I wanted to enter the field of medicine. I was told this was cliché and unrealistic and that it is seen by every admission's officer in every PA school in the country every year. Unfortunately for me, it is also true. Borne out of an unrelenting sense of curiosity and a drive to have every "why" and "how" answered I naturally gravitated to a field where there is never a shortage of whys and how's. Fortunately for everyone involved, instead of an essay about my passion for chemistry and human physiology, I hope to share, not necessarily my motivations to enter the medical field, but fundamentally what kind of care provider I want to be and why the role of physician assistant is right for me.

I have to admit that I got off to a rocky start. When I first started work as a nurse aide in a retirement community I expected to hate my job. I thought that I would be able to grin and bear it while I racked up my clinical hours and then be welcomed into PA school with open arms and be able forget what the acronym "BM" stood for. However, I am not above admitting when I am wrong and I have never been happier to be wrong than I was in this instance. I quickly realized that I was doing both my residents and myself an injustice by thinking myself above the task of helping the unstable resident with Parkinson's disease get her shower or helping the resident with macular degeneration change the batteries in his hearing aids. And when I had my first experience with a resident who had fallen I was brought back to moment at university and a lesson that I should never have forgotten.

During my sophomore year, I joined an organization called Community Emergency Response Team (CERT). In CERT, a small group of students like me were trained to perform search and rescue, basic triage, and assistance for other emergency management officials. During one such training session meant to simulate a collapsed building, I found my way through the dark hallways of the "collapsed" building and found myself in front of Hannah, a "patient." I quickly assessed Hannah's injuries with a couple of simple questions and decided that she warranted a yellow triage tag. I proudly put the tag on her wrist and was about to move on to the next patient when one of the CERT leaders asked me a question that stopped me in my tracks: "Is that really all you're going to do for this patient?" I realized then that I while I had executed the science of triage flawlessly, I'd left out the most important part: I had quite literally forgotten to care for the patient. Although it seems so simple and obvious to me now, that question brought to the forefront that caring for patients is more than applying the science I have learned in the classroom and certainly more than breezing through my clinical hour requirement with no regard for the reason it is a requirement in the first place. Knowledge of scientific processes and performing skills from a checklist are only the start in giving my patients the care they want, need, and deserve.

It is surprising that I didn't remember Hannah when I started my job as a nurse aide because it was my moment with her that led me away from a major in biochemistry, my favorite subject, and toward public health. My public health classes shaped my personal philosophy that healthcare is a right, not a privilege granted to a few. It was, in fact, my public health studies that drove me to consider a career as a PA instead of as an MD, which I had originally intended, since as a PA, I can fill an important void in our current healthcare system.

I'd like to think that I've come a long way since that evening spent with Hannah on the floor of a dark classroom and that I've come even further during my time as a CNA. Being a CNA in a retirement community was not my first choice in obtaining my clinical hours. I had imagined myself doing something slightly more glamorous, or at least played o my scientific strengths, like working as a medical assistant in a surgeon's office. In retrospect, however, being a CNA was exactly the experience I needed. I have found emotional maturity in my interactions with my residents, many of whom I will be in contact with for years to come simply because I enjoy them as people, not just as patients. This is the kind of clinician I plan to be. I want to be a care provider who not only understands the whys and hows, but goes a step further. Hannah, just like my fallen resident, needed empathy. Sometimes my residents need reassurance, sometimes they need a helping hand, and often they need one of medicine's most proven panaceas: a good laugh.

Commentary Essay 53

I really like this essay. It's unique, honest, revealing, and fun/interesting to read. Of course, I still have a few comments.

My biggest comment is that you say in your opening paragraph that you'll explain why being a PA is the right profession for you, yet you don't. Yes, you mention your public health classes, but not really anything else. You could stay a CNA or be an RN. Why couldn't you be an MD with an interest in public health? One of the most important things about writing anything is to honor the promise you make in your opening paragraph!

Most of my other suggestions are picky. "I have to admit that I got off to a rocky start" could be more concise — "I admit I got off to a rocky start." You can omit the fourth sentence in that paragraph. Read your essay out loud and see where you stumble on long sentences. There are a few. See if you really need everything or there are redundancies. Every sentence should make a new point. Remember, your readers are seeing thousands of essays. Make it easy for them to love yours.

Overall, excellent work.

Essay 54

Around the age of seven my family and I moved to the United States from Iran. Around that time my grandfather, who was already here, had a stroke and was in and out of hospitals and doctor offices. I attended those visits with him and my father and, even though I was young and barely spoke English, I was still able to notice the quality of care that my grandfather was provided by the healthcare professionals. I was very intrigued by how the doctors and nurses took such good care of him and just like any young child, I walked around and I would proudly say that I would become a doctor one day!

I knew at a young age I wanted to work in some kind of health career. Throughout my adolescence I was always attracted to science courses and I would excel in them. I took many health related courses in high school and was privileged to take an Allied Health class where I, along with other students, was able to volunteer in nursing homes and shadow different departments within our local hospital. That was an eye opening experience and it reassured my passion for the health profession. However, it wasn't until my freshman year of college that I was introduced to the Physician Assistant field. During my undergraduate at the University of North Carolina at Greensboro (UNCG) I majored in Biology where I took a keen interest into the human based biology courses such Human Anatomy, Cellular Biology, and Biochemistry. I am still very intrigued by how the human body works and even though some concepts are difficult to understand, I am always eager to learn more. I attended many seminars during my undergrad at UNCG about the different careers within the health field, and each time the prospect of becoming a Physician Assistant became more and more appealing!

Within the past two years, I was fortunate enough to acquire a job with a company that provides in-home care for people with disabilities. I was placed with a 13-year-old with Rhett's Syndrome. My job allowed me to provide assistance with the client's everyday routines, such as, aiding with toileting, feeding, showering, and walking. I also worked on specific goals to better the clients cognitive and motor skills. I have gained so much experience from working, more than I could have ever imagined. I have learned so much about myself including the amount of patience and commitment I have to help accommodate her life and make activities of daily living easier on her. Since the client is not able to communicate verbally, I have learned how to depend on other factors such as body language, recognition of differences in her mood from day to day, and coming up with alternate ways to communicate. I have learned what it takes to deal with a person who depends on you for everything, similar to how a patient coming in for a visit depends on their PA for the correct diagnosis and the right treatment. I continue to learn more and more each day I work with her.

Another experience that has helped motivate me to become a PA has been the opportunity to shadow an actual Physician Assistant. I was able to observe the PA interact with her patients and perform examinations. I have gained a lot from that experience. I learned how to interact with different types of patients and I noticed that it takes a lot more than being knowledgeable in medicine to be an effective health provider. Apart from the typical roles of a PA, I learned from my shadowing experience that a PA needs to be attentive, amicable, and possess interpersonal skills.

Throughout my career as a student and a caregiver, I have learned that along with my alacrity for medicine, I possess qualities that would enhance my role as a Physician Assistant. Most importantly I am a good listener, a quality that is significant in any health profession. I am compassionate for others, and possess a lot of patience. I am prepared to work hard to be the best

Physician Assistant I can be, and I look forward for the opportunity to begin the next chapter of my life.

Commentary Essay 54

You have a lot of great experience and good writing skills, things many applicants lack. That's gives you a definite edge. However, there are ways to tighten your essay and really make it shine.

You don't need the first paragraph at all. It's so remote in time and such a common occurrence (yes, even moving to the U.S. from Iran or another country, and especially experiences with ailing grandparents), that it's not remarkable enough to include.

The second paragraph is good, but it has a lot of extra words (and a couple used improperly) that make it bulky. By the way, never use exclamation points, and the word "passion" is so overused, it doesn't mean much to Admissions Directors. Take a look at these edited sentences and see if you miss anything:

"I knew at a young age I wanted to work in healthcare. During high school, I excelled in science, and was privileged to take an Allied Health class where students volunteered in nursing homes and shadowed different departments at our local hospital. That was an eye opening experience and reinforced my interest in medicine. As an undergraduate I majored in Biology, where I took a keen interest into the human-based biology courses. While a freshman, I was introduced to the physician assistant field. I had attended many seminars about the different careers within healthcare, and each time the prospect of a career as a physician assistant became more appealing."

What I really wanted to know after I read that paragraph is why the prospect of becoming a PA appealed. You didn't say and you should. Admissions Directors want to know specifically why you're choosing the PA profession.

Read your other paragraphs carefully, and see where you've written more than needed. You'll find words to eliminate, I'm sure.

You do a good job of writing about your experience with your patient. Maybe in your PA shadowing experience a particular case stands out as an example of exemplary PA work. You could write about that.

In your final paragraph, the word alacrity isn't the best choice. You want to emphasize ability, not eagerness.

Essay 55

Every Sunday was innocent, youthful bliss at grandma's house after church. You never imagine the day when that house would no longer be grandma's house, the place to meet up after church and run around with all of your cousins, the day your big, tight knit family loses the glue that held everyone together.

My grandmother was the epicenter of our large Irish catholic family and every holiday, birthday, and celebration was centered at her house. Most of childhood family memories come from being at her house, including the memory of her smoking one cigarette after another. My cousins and I used to hide her cigarettes every time we visited because we wanted her to stop in the sincerest way. Her habits caught up to her and brought with them great illness and eventually lung cancer. We moved her into our home so she could have constant care and comfort of being with her own family. As a senior in high school, I used to do my homework by her bedside just so I could spend time with her. I watched her waste away before my eyes and wished so badly that there was something I could have done differently to save her and at the same time I wanted to still do something to

change what was inevitable. One day we as the entire family huddled around her bed, we watched her gasp her last breath. That
was the last time our entire family was together, seven years ago.

I had always had a keen interest in science and the human body,
but that was the moment I knew I had to do what I could to heal
others. It's so much more than making someone well again, it's
keep families together and allowing the opportunity to create
new memories.

Commentary Essay 55

It's a rare essay that requires more, but yours is one. It's really only
begun.

After reading this, Admissions Directors will only know that you
have a loving family, an interest in science and the human body,
and want to help other people. That's not enough.

Why are you applying to PA school? Have you shadowed a PA?
Worked in any area of healthcare? Done any volunteer work, health
related or not? Even if you don't have experience in healthcare, you
need to provide good reasons for a PA school to consider you.

Take a look at the other essays posted here and read the comments.
It may help you get an idea of what schools expect to see in an essay.

Essay 56

It's not every day that I find myself in a children's hospital, let
alone the Offenbach Kinderklinik in Germany; however, on May
2, 2006, I was there to perform with BYU's Living Legends. The

group is made up of Latin, Polynesian and Native American dancers, and I was there to perform a "Native American Grass Dance." Gathered around, was the media, the attending physician, medical staff, and of course the children. I hoped to help bring smiles and entertainment to the audience and share my culture, but what I didn't expect was what they would share with me in turn. As I danced to the rhythm of native drums and song, I couldn't help but notice the children's reactions. They truly looked at us with the most beautiful smiles. Their laughter was universal, and their applause was genuine. What I hadn't noticed, were the burns on their bodies, and the scars both physical and mental left behind from a war in Iraq. After our performance, the attending physician explained how inspiring its message of love and unity was for the children. We represented three very different cultures united in a love for life. He further explained that the children were casualties and innocent bystanders in a conflict that did not represent such a thing. I had paid attention to what the media was saying back home in the states about the war, but this was real, and the children were real. Regardless of politics, religion, or any other belief I looked at them and knew they were all part of the human family. As I looked inward, I knew in my heart that I wanted to help others despite their background. It was in this moment I realized I wanted to do all that I can to protect, sustain, and improve the physical and mental wellbeing of every individual I served.

Upon returning from tour I served a two year proselytizing mission for my church in New Jersey, and was called to do so in Spanish. Though in my eyes, I went to do a service for the Latinos in that state, I left having been served by them. They welcomed me into their homes and shared with me their foods, music, and love of life. It was this love of life that many of them struggled to sustain, especially when it came to their health. During service opportunities every week, like translating, I saw some of their struggles to even obtain basic medical care. Had I not been around them, I would have never understood the complexities of being an immigrant in an inner city, while seeking such care. I did not feel that it should be this way, so when I finished my mission and started school again I switched my degree from music to the sciences. This way, I could pursue a profession in the medical field and help make a change.

I gained a lot of knowledge during my education, and I also learned a lot about life and myself. At one point I was struggling with a genetics class due to illness and surgery. I finally had to ask myself if I was willing to do what was necessary to pass the class. I was! I learned to really study, focus, and sacrifice as I finally passed. That experience has now empowered me in my professional work to continue my education as a lifelong learner apart from what's going on in my life. While in school, the knowledge I sought wasn't just about the sciences, but I also wanted more life experiences. I have since traveled the world to many other countries with Living Legends, even representing the group as its president. In preparation for our tours we studied the cultures, language, and history so that we might better connect with our audiences. As we continued to do outreaches to hospitals, orphanages, and schools I found myself falling more in love with the people. That love has since carried over to the patients I have served.

While working with the mentally disabled, those in Hospice, and children in Head Start, I have seen the struggles that each at risk population faces, and how they need medical providers that are willing to be advocates on their behalf. I have also seen the need for committed medical professionals on the reservations I have danced at, and in the inner cities that I have proselytized in. My experiences overall have truly cemented within my heart that I want to be that committed caretaker and advocate. It was through shadowing that I decided that becoming a Physician Assistant (PA) is what best suited me, and would enable me to accomplish these desires. I know that to work as a PA, within a family practice, would be the most fulfilling for me while practicing in any medically underserved and rural community. It is in these areas that I know my love for people and cultures, and passion to be an advocate for certain populations, would be best used. It is my hope, that when I become a PA, that I can lift the people up with me, just as I had sang so many times before in Living Legends. "Go my son, go and climb the ladder...From on the ladder of an education you can see to help your Indian Nation. Then reach, my son, and lift your people up with you.

Commentary Essay 56

You've certainly accomplished much already. Your compassion and dedication to helping people is evident, and your future patients will benefit greatly.

The essay, though, focuses too much on your Living Legends and mission work. I'll show you a couple of places to cut some of that to leave room to write about your health care related work — hospice, working with those who are mentally disabled, and shadowing. Those are what the Admissions Directors and personnel will want to know more about. Put some of the emotion you express in your writing about Living Legends toward examples of work with actual patients. It will ground your essay in the reality of life as a health care provider.

You also haven't said why you want to be a PA as opposed to other professions within medicine. You'll need to do that, and one of the best ways is to use a PA/patient case as an example. What did the PA do that impressed you? How was the PA different than other health care providers?

Please never use exclamation points. Your written words should make the point.

Take a look at these edited sentences:

"It's not every day that I find myself in a children's hospital, let alone the Offenbach Kinderklinik in Germany; however, on May 2, 2006, I was there to perform with BYU's Living Legends. Gathered around was the media, the attending physician, medical staff, and of course, the children. I hoped to help bring smiles and entertainment to the audience and share my culture, but what I didn't expect was what they would share with me in turn. As I danced I couldn't help but notice the children's beautiful smiles. What I hadn't noticed, were the burns on their bodies, and the scars both physical and mental left behind from a war in Iraq."

"Upon returning from tour I served a mission for my church in New Jersey, and was called to do so in Spanish. Though in my eyes, I went to do a service for the Latinos in that state, I left having been served by them. They shared with me their foods, music, and love of life. It was this love of life that many of them struggled to sustain, especially when it came to their health. I saw their struggles to even obtain basic medical care. I learned the complexities of being an immigrant in an inner city seeking such care."

Those are just two examples. You could and should do the same with every paragraph. This will leave you space to add the important information.

Essay 57

I was sitting on a confining wooden chair in a small hovel surrounded by nursing students conducting a home visit. In front of us was sitting Jane Doe, a 25-year-old patient from the clinic where I volunteered in a remote village in Guatemala. She was explaining to us how she had contracted HIV and how difficult it was to be under medical treatment while supporting her two fatherless children. Then I asked her was if the people in her village knew about her disease: "They would curse me, humiliate my family, and kick us out of the neighborhood if they found out that I have AIDS!" she exclaimed in a Spanish with a Mayan accent. She told us that she had almost died two years before when she acquired tuberculosis and her worst fear was that one day she would be too sick to take care of her children and mother. We listened to her, educated her about the importance of adhering to her HIV medications, and prayed together for her wellbeing. We also helped her children with their homework and gave the family some donations we had collected. The following week, Jane brought her kids to the clinic because they were sick. Because of the low quality public health system in the town, they waited almost four hours to see the doctor and one hour to obtain their prescription. I was helping in the pharmacy and when I gave Jane the medications she smiled, said "Gracias!", and gave me a big hug.

Growing up in a small town in Mexico, I experienced a similar healthcare system. Every time I was sick, I would have to spend hours at the clinic waiting for the doctor to see me for only a few minutes. The medicine prescribed was always a very painful penicillin injection for a wide range of illnesses, but mostly for common colds. If that was unavailable, then I would get an Ampicillin shot which would be even more painful that I was unable to walk for hours. That was when my idea of becoming a clinician emerged. I knew there were ill people around the world waiting a long time to see a doctor and I could do something about it. After meticulous research on different health care professions during my undergraduate studies, I found physician assistant

(PA) to be the career for me. As a PA, I will be able to balance medicine practice and patient care reducing the time patients have to spend in the waiting room. Faster care means less pain and patients are inclined to come to their appointments and build strong bonds with their providers.

From my work and volunteer experiences, I learned that it is imperative to establish deep relationships with patients to gain their trust and provide the proper care. As a PA, I will create these bonds with my patients similarly to what I have observed in all the PAs who I have shadowed in different specialties. Jane is seen at her clinic in Guatemala frequently and I have constant communication with her doctor about Jane's condition. I have also presented this case to doctors at The Institute of Human Virology (IHV) at University of Maryland, School of Medicine where I work as a clinical research coordinator and they will advise on Jane's medical intervention if necessary. The IHV is an archetype of institutions dedicated to serve the needs of the medically underserved communities. Our patients also share their stories with me when they come to the clinic for their followup visits, and unlike Jane, they have learned to overcome the extant stigma in our country. More importantly, they have the medical and moral support of healthcare providers, partners, friends, families, and the community. Unfortunately, there are many people who are oblivious to having serious medical conditions and need treatment. I want to concentrate on serving these communities by providing diagnosis, treatment, and education.

My current job is very rewarding and I have the pleasure of working directly under the supervision physicians from whom I learn extensively. I interact with patients with various health conditions who often ask me for medical advice but I am unable to assist them any further. When I become a PA, I will have the training and confidence to provide more service to our society as a healthcare provider. I will also enjoy lifelong learning since there will always be new ways medicine can improve life. I strongly believe that my past personal, work, and academic experiences have prepared me for the rigorous PA education your institution offers. I am prepared to dedicate my life to being physician assistant.

Commentary Essay 57

You have an impressive resume and have chronicled it very well. You did an excellent job with just a couple of words — "confining wooden chair in a small hovel" of describing Jane Doe's living conditions.

Of course, I still have suggestions, including a couple of grammar/writing tips. First, when you include dialog, preface it with a comma, not a colon. You don't need to explain that PA is the acronym for physician assistant.

Whenever you have the opportunity to use active verbs, take it. For example, here's a stronger way to write your opening two sentences:

"I sat on a confining wooden chair in a small hovel surrounded by nursing students conducting a home visit. We listened to Jane Doe, a 25-year old patient from the clinic where I volunteered in a remote village in Guatemala. She explained how she had contracted HIV, and how difficult it was to support her two fatherless children while undergoing treatment."

You could leave out some details about your work with Jane and your childhood experiences to write more about your shadowing experiences. Omit the information about Jane's children entirely. It's wonderful that you helped them with their homework, but that information doesn't add anything here. As to their health care, when you talk about your own experiences as a child, you've made the point. It's like repeating a car chase scene in a movie. You don't need more than one. In fact, there are many places to cut or shorten sentences because you've made your point already. Read your essay carefully and be ruthless about taking out unnecessary words. There are many.

Your sentence starting with "After meticulous research" should be the start of a new paragraph. (I'm not sure if the formatting on the website changed your paragraphs, but they should be shorter rather than longer. Start a new one with "Jane is seen regularly," too). Then add more detail about why you want to be a PA as opposed to another field. Why not be an MD?

I love the way you tied your current job's limitations to your goal of becoming a PA. That's excellent.

You have a great start. All you need is a careful edit and a few additional sentences about your shadowing experiences to help your readers understand why the PA profession is for you.

Essay 58

The patient was a 8 year old boy, dizzy, scared, and angry. His hearing aids weren't working for him and the world was a cacophony of distorted sounds that made him unwilling to spend time communicating with his family, teachers, and friends. But on this day his physician assistant kneeled down to his eye level, and communicated with him slowly, by writing his thoughts on paper and by mouthing his words so the patient could understand, to ask what was wrong. The physician assistant made the patient feel safe through his clinical empathy and bedside manner. His treatment helped the patient get better and feel happier.

The patient was me. The physician assistant was Danny Kamlet. Danny had no way to understand the chilled isolation I felt as a hearing impaired youth; when I desperately wanted to hear the joke everyone laughed at, the teacher's explanation for the math problem on the board, or to flirt with the cute girl. Teachers had said I was a poor student when the reality was that I couldn't read their lips and understand them as they faced the blackboard and lectured. Many of my hearing disabled peers, unfortunately, didn't graduate high school or college but I persevered due to the compassion, communication, and resourcefulness of my mother and health care providers like Danny.

My mother supported my deaf brother and me by herself; if one of our hearing aids broke, she took out mortgages on her house so that we could get another one. She read with us every night to help us learn what we didn't in school, instilling in me an appreciation for hard work and education so I could thrive. I learned to compensate by studying with other students, and communicating with my teachers so that I can excel in my courses.

Danny and other health care providers helped change my life for the better through empathetic communication in addition to their medical knowledge. A few years ago, after I finished my sophomore year of college, my doctor and audiologist helped me receive financial support to get cochlear implants that have greatly improved my hearing and quality of life. After college, my physician assistant Michael Johnson used his inquisition in a general checkup to find that I was losing eyebrow hair and was consistently fatigued. He surmised that I might have hypothyroidism and low vitamin D blood levels and subsequent tests confirmed this to be true. His prescription of Levothyroxin and my supplementation of vitamin D have helped to improve my energy, mental acuity, and metabolism.

Because of my amazing health care providers, I've grown so much as a person and student in recent years. With my improved hearing, I've taken up new hobbies that I previously would have avoided, such as blues dancing. In the 47 credits I've completed after receiving treatment for hypothyroidism and upgrading my cochlear processors, I've excelled with a GPA of 3.76. I owe so much of my improvement to the care of my physician assistants.

In the model of compassionate giving set by my health care providers, I've tried to live my life doing what I can to help those that are less privileged. I've helped other deaf people get disability benefits so they can afford critical equipment upgrades. I spent time in college baking bread for the abused women of Safe Harbor through a group called Baked Benevolence. I asked my friends to give my twenty-first birthday gifts to my runathon effort at my college, and raised over 200 dollars for abused children of Knox County. I will never completely understand the gamut of emotions that abused children and women have gone through but I empathize with them having uncertain health and understand how to communicate and help them. By contributing to their lives, I found fulfillment as a member of a healthy community; treating individuals of all backgrounds with respect and grace.

This is why I want to be a physician assistant! I want to communicate and empathize to help the scared and confused patient feel safe and informed. I want to give comprehensive examinations that get to the root of each symptom and communicate how to afford and administer treatment. I want to help underserved populations receive the full extent of health benefits possible. As someone who overcame a disability through excellent health care, I dream of helping other underserved populations receive the best health care possible.

Commentary Essay 58

The opening two paragraphs of your essay are excellent. They grabbed my attention immediately, and made me want to keep reading. That's your goal!

You could eliminate a few words to make the sentences flow better. For example, here's a revised sentence.

"His hearing aids weren't working for him and the world was a cacophony of distorted sounds that made him unwilling to communicate with his family, teachers, and friends. But on this day, his physician assistant kneeled to eye level and communicated slowly, by writing his thoughts and mouthing his words so the patient could understand. The physician assistant made the patient feel safe through his empathy and bedside manner. His treatment helped the patient get better and feel happier."

I'm guessing you won't miss any of the deleted words.

You don't need the third paragraph at all.

It's lucky that you have such a wonderful mom, but the information about her doesn't help the Admissions folks know you better. Omit it and use the space to elaborate on your qualities and skills.

The problem continues in the fourth paragraph.

It's good to explain that health issues impacted your grades (Admissions Directors want to know why they weren't good), but the details aren't necessary.

Take this revised sentence for example: "After College, my physician assistant Michael Johnson used his intuition and skills to discover I suffered from hypothyroidism. His diagnosis and treatment have helped to improve my energy, mental acuity, and metabolism." It says everything the reader needs to know.

While it's great that you do amazing volunteer work, you'll need to explain how those experiences contribute to the skill set you'll need as a PA.

Delete many of the details and focus on things akin to your statement: "I will never completely understand the gamut of emotions that abused children and women have gone through, but I empathize with them having uncertain health and understand how to communicate and help them. By contributing to their lives, I found fulfillment as a member of a healthy community; treating individuals of all backgrounds with respect and grace, treating individuals of all backgrounds with respect and grace."

Your ability to empathize and communicate with those less fortunate is well established.

What else have you learned? Has the volunteer work increased your leadership or decision-making skills? Your ability to work as part of a team? Have you needed to remain calm when shelter clients are upset?

I'm assuming you don't have a job or shadowing experience in the medical field because it's not in your essay, so you'll need to beef up skills you've acquired in other aspects of your life.

What you also need to do is explain more specifically why you want to be a PA.

There are a million things you could do to help people in the way you mention in your last paragraph — many in the medical profession. Why not be a nurse or a doctor?

Your job is to convince the admissions folks that being a PA is the only option that interests you, and to show that you have much to offer their program.

Go back through your essay and scrutinize every sentence. Does it help Admissions Directors and faculty know something new about you? If it doesn't, out it goes.

By the way, ditch the exclamation point. Never use them in essays. Your words should be the exclamation point.

Essay 59

I woke up with a tube down my throat, unable to speak, over-whelmed by voices all repeatedly saying my name. Over all of them I heard my mom, "Lindsay, squeeze my hand if you can hear me", so I did, but that's where the memory ends. That's where a week in the ICU and road to recovery began. I would come to learn that I had suffered a heat stroke while running a half marathon on a scorching July morning and my organs be-gan to shut down. Although it was one of the more difficult times in my life, it was also one of the most important, as it helped so-lidify my desire to become a Physician Assistant and to change lives like one doctor changed mine.

Long before my accident, I had the opportunity to shadow an Orthopedic Trauma Surgeon. Over the years, I've gone into the operating room with him dozens of time, compiling hundreds of hours, but I will never forget the very first surgery I saw. It was a middle-aged man undergoing an ORIF of his fractured hu-merus. For the surgeons, it was a run-of-the-mill surgery, just another Monday. But for me, it was the first day of the rest of my life. A wide-eyed 18year old surrounded by blue sterile fields, drills and screws, I knew where I wanted to direct my life. That was when I decided that a career in the medical field was the only option for me. During numerous visits to the OR, I watched the attending surgeon, the residents, the PA and the nurses. The way they worked together reminded me of my high school track team when we ran a relay race, they passed the tools between mem-bers, each doing some of the work to achieve a common goal. At this point, I was not entirely sure what a PA did. The more I ob-served, the more I began to notice that the PA is a crucial part to the relay team; an extension of the team of doctors. The doctors pass the PA the baton and they shoulder some of the work so that as doctors they can focus on their specialties. It allows the entire relay team to reach their goals and creates the safest, most effective approach to patient care. Much like being a part of the 4x800m relay team, I could see myself fitting in to the medical relay team as the PA, the middle leg, the extension between the doctors and the finish line of helping the patient.

Following my heat stroke was a weeklong stint in the ICU at Columbia St. Mary's Hospital. During this time I was scared, sad, confused, defeated. My organs had begun to fail and were slowly recovering, which left me exhausted. I could barely stand, let alone walk, and had more lines in me than I could count. One doctor helped me through it all. Dr. Stepke, a gastroenterologist, was at my bedside every day, as my liver had the worst injury. Not only did he provide me with extraordinary medical care, but with the mental and emotional support that I needed. I was told I would be on bed rest for six weeks and limited physical activity for six weeks after that. For a runner, this was awful. The compassion and empathy that Dr. Stepke had for me soars above any other health care worker I've ever come across. I was 19, in the hospital, scared, and he made me feel like everything was going to be okay, like he truly cared for me and that he understood how I was feeling. I followed up with Dr. Stepke weekly for six weeks and he never wavered in his support during my recovery. There is something so invaluable about learning first hand the effects that your potential career can have on someone. My relationship with Dr. Stepke was another reassurance that I was meant to be a PA. Since then, every step of the way on my journey towards becoming a PA, I have always strived to make every patient feel how he made me feel: supported, cared for, and understood.

In more than two years working as a CNA, there is one patient that stands out. Her name was Laura, a 37yearold admitted with a GI bleed. Laura was an alcoholic with dozens of medical problems stemming from her drinking and I would quickly come to realize that she was nearing the end of her short life. Suddenly her care became so much more than the medicine. I cared for her mentally and emotionally, as Dr. Stepke had done for me, while she slowly accepted what was going to happen, while she and the Child Life Specialist told her two young sons, while she was no longer able to walk on her own. This was the hardest time in her life. She was defeated, depressed, dying. After two weeks of working with Laura almost every day, she was discharged. Laura died two days later in the comfort of her home surrounded by family. In my time with her, I did my best to provide her with the empathy and compassion that I had once felt from Dr. Stepke. In my time as a CNA, I've learned communication, working as a cohesive team, patience and improvisation, but working with Laura taught me so much more. Through her, I learned about the importance of holistic medicine, in taking care of the mind, body and soul. This can best be achieved by working together as healthcare professionals, passing the baton and ultimately crossing the finish line as a team.

First, I observed and saw I wanted to be a Physician Assistant. Then, I was the patient and felt that I wanted to be a Physician Assistant. Once I felt the impact an incredible doctor can have on a person, I adopted those practices into my own role as a CNA. And once the two came together, working as a team to care for someone in such a vulnerable state, like I had once been, I saw the rest of my life unfold as a Physician Assistant.

Commentary Essay 59

This is an excellent start to your personal statement. Your descriptions are vivid — I can picture you perfectly in the ICU, and that's exactly what you want your readers to do.

In the third paragraph you lose your focus. The goal is to let Admissions Directors and faculty know why you want to be a PA. When I read this, I saw no connection between your interactions with Dr. Stepke and wanting to be a PA, other than he showed unwavering support. Why did your relationship with the doctor make you want to be a PA? You never say and you need to. Why not be a doctor instead? Compassion and support is a small part of a PA's job. You could omit most of that paragraph and just use the following:

"Following my heat stroke was a weeklong stint in the ICU at Columbia St. Mary's Hospital. One doctor helped me through it all. Dr. Stepke, a gastroenterologist, was at my bedside every day, as my liver had the worst injury. Not only did he provide me with extraordinary medical care, but with the mental and emotional support that I needed. Since then, every step of the way on my journey towards becoming a PA, I have always strived to make every patient feel how he made me feel: supported, cared for, and understood."

In your paragraph about Laura (which overall was excellent) omit the references to Dr. Stepke. You don't need them. This sentence would then read: "Suddenly her care became so much more than the medicine. I cared for her mentally and emotionally." Leave this sentence out completely: "In my time with her, I did my best to provide her with the empathy and compassion that I had once felt from Dr. Stepke." It's redundant for one.

Use the extra space to reinforce why you've chosen to pursue the PA profession as opposed to any other. Then you'll be able to make your conclusion stronger. It's weak as it stands now. Saying that you "felt" you wanted to be a PA isn't compelling.

Essay 60

I was sitting in the examination room of the cardiology office with tears slowly streaming down. My father could read the sign of disappointment on my face as the cardiologist briefly explains my EKG results with what seemed as indifference to my situation. At the age of 15 a cardiologist diagnosed me with a heart condition called as Lown–Ganong–Levine syndrome. However, the cardiologist was not completely certain as to the causation of my irregular heartbeat and referred me to a specialized cardiologist. Being an athletic girl who played soccer at an extremely competitive level I was perplexed as to why I was unexpectedly experiencing these alarming symptoms due to an irregular and very rapid heartbeat. Multiple procedures and four cardiologists later I was forced to retire from competitive soccer and left without answers. The most frustrating part of this entire process is what seemed as the lack of compassion and empathy from these doctors. I was left heartbroken with responses like "Just stop playing soccer if that's when your heart bothers you" and "maybe you should find a new hobby". This feeling of disappointment from the insensitive doctors made me realize I want to be a person who provides admirable healthcare to patients in a caring way. Through my experiences and also investing time job shadowing a physician assistant (PA) and doctor have further solidified my desire to become a PA. A doctor and PA are both knowledgeable, but a PA is able to spend more quality time with the patient as opposed to a doctor who is on a strict schedule because their time is very valuable. This additional time allows the PA to interact with patient and gain the patient's trust.

When I was 19 years old I taught myself the foundation to medicine by becoming a certified and registered pharmacy technician. Over the past 6 years I have worked in various pharmacy settings ranging from retail to hospital positions. By excelling at my job and taking the extra steps to absorb as much knowledge as possible, I can interpret sigs on prescriptions, know which medications are used for specific therapies, understand how medications should be taken for optimum results, and fully grasp the process insurance companies use to cover medications. As a PA I will be able to exercise this information by providing accurate and speedy care. Knowing that a patient must first try Omeprazole before prescribing Nexium in order for the insurance company to cover Nexium allows the patient to quickly treat their GERD without wasting valuable time. Currently, I work for a company that provides medications, durable medical equipment, and skilled nursing and rehabilitative care to medically fragile infants and children. We care for children that are genetically born with a defect, which impairs their ability to ingest or digest food. Others are born without congenital defects, but experience a traumatic event, such as a near drowning experience or tragic car accident, which leaves them with debilitated. I may not directly interact with these children on a daily basis, but seeing their faces light up when I do justify all the care, precision, and hard work I put into my job. This gratification motivates me to further my career in the healthcare field and become a PA so that I am able to provide more direct patient care and see these smiling faces on a daily basis.

Not only has my work experience proved that I'm ready to dedicate myself toward becoming a PA, but my schoolwork has as well. When I first started college I can honestly say I wasn't mentally ready due to a lack of focus. I placed more emphasis on trivial things, like hanging out with my friends instead of studying. It was uncharacteristic of me to be failing classes, as I was the girl who graduated high school 23rd in a class of 900 students because of my 4.1 GPA. I lost sight of my goals in the beginning of college and soon realized my priorities. After my realization, I spent dramatically less time with my friends and more time with my books. Managing my time and taking the proper amount of time to prepare for my tests improved my grades.

Although I adore being a pharmacy technician, it hasn't fulfilled my need for patient care. I want to participate more directly than I currently can, I want to be much more hands on. With that being said, I would like to step out of the background and move towards the forefront of patient care. I want to be the person with the proper skill sets and medical knowledge so that I can help others live a life of the highest quality possible. As a PA there's a choice of many career paths ranging from assisting in surgery to working in a pediatric office. Therefore, becoming a PA opens countless doors and opportunities for intellectual, personal, and professional growth, while simultaneously serving the needs of others. Becoming a PA is exactly the path for me.

Commentary Essay 60

If there's anything positive to say about your diagnosis at age 15, it's the tremendous insight it gave you about the medical profession. You're smart to open your essay that way. The other things you write about are good, too. It's important to explain why your grades weren't great, and to talk about your adult experiences. This is a very good start to your statement.

I say good start because there are some issues. Some are grammatical, such as using past tense and present tense in the same few sentences, and placing quotation marks inside of punctuation.

Other examples — writing the singular word doctor and then referring to the doctor as "their," and saying "foundation to" instead of "foundation of." Although these are fairly minor errors and very common, when I interviewed Admissions Directors and faculty, all said grammar errors could be fatal to the application.

There are two ways to really make your essay shine. One is structure and the second is content.

Structurally, you'd move the section about your shadowing experiences from the first paragraph to a new third paragraph. You'll have to change some of the way you've written your essay to make it work, but that's part of the process.

As to content, you'd shorten your first paragraph (I'll show you below) and use the extra space to write about your shadowing experiences. You'll do this for two reasons. One, every person from admissions I spoke with said, "Keep your personal story short. A few sentences is enough. Secondly, you want to show your readers that you know what it takes to do the job, and then tie your skills to some of those requirements. I'm not talking about making a list of PA job duties, but rather to describe a case or an overview of what you learned by shadowing, and how some of your personal skills (not clinical as you've already done that when describing your pharmacy work) fit in with the profession. Take out the "therefore" in your conclusion. It takes away from the strength of your sentence.

Here's the edited first paragraph, which is now two paragraphs. Notice that the first section is in present tense. It makes it real and compelling despite the lapse in time:

"I'm sitting in the examination room of the cardiology office with tears slowly streaming. My father could read the sign of disappointment on my face as the cardiologist briefly explains my EKG results with what seems as indifference to my situation. At the age of 15 I am diagnosed with a heart condition called as Lown–Ganong–Levine syndrome.

Multiple procedures and four cardiologists later, I was forced to retire from competitive soccer and left without answers. The most frustrating part of this entire process was the lack of compassion and empathy from doctors who said, "Just stop playing soccer if that's when your heart bothers you" and "Maybe you should find a new hobby." This insensitivity made me realize I want to be a person who provides admirable healthcare to patients in a caring way."

Look at your essay and see where you have extra words. There are many of them. Cut ruthlessly to make your essay as concise as possible and focused on the essentials.

Essay 61

In my sophomore year of high school I met the woman who would ultimately spark my interest in pursuing a career in the medical field. Liz was the new athletic trainer at my school and I was the manager of the boys' soccer team. We developed a great relationship from the first day we met, and I soon became the student athletic trainer. Every day during last period I would go to her office and she would teach me about sports injuries, proper wrapping techniques, and how to rehabilitate specific injuries. I became intrigued with the athletic training career, and by the time junior year came, I knew that was what I wanted to do for the rest of my life. Unfortunately, that same year Liz was not rehired, and I realized there was not much job security with that career. I knew I still wanted to work in the medical field though, so I began researching different options with my guidance counselor at school, and that was when we came across the physician assistant profession.

Once we began researching about PAs more, I really began to envision my future. Though I had never realized it, I have seen a PA since the time I was a baby. She always takes the time to talk to me, help me, and give me the best care she can, even if it is just for something as simple as a cold or an ear infection. On the rare occasion that I have to see the doctor in the office, though he too gives the best care he can, the visit always seems less personal. I believe that is one of the things that really drew me into pursuing this career – having the ability to develop great patient provider relationships. I also learned that my little sister goes to school with a girl whose mother is a PA as well. Speaking with her and hearing how much she loved her job only made me want to be a PA even more.

Another thing that really interested me about PAs was the team dynamic between them and physicians. I like the idea of being able to have independence, while also having the physician to fall back on when help is needed. The trust within the team is something I believe is of utmost importance. I have had the great opportunity of being able to work as a clinical assistant in an occupational medicine office for the last year during college breaks. This was my first job in health care, and I was excited to finally get to see that team dynamic play out. Watching the PA, as well as the nurse practitioner, and the doctors all interact was very interesting to me.

Working in the occupational medicine office has given me the chance to learn some basic medical procedures. I was taught how to clean and stitch, or glue, small lacerations, how to irrigate an eye to flush out foreign bodies, and also how to examine an eye for foreign bodies. The people who taught me these things were the PA and the CRNP. I noticed that they were the most willing of all the people in the office to teach me new things, rather than just pass me by as another assistant. Them taking the time to teach me only further excited me to hopefully be able to be in a position to do that for other people later in life. I also noticed that our PA really took the time to explain his diagnoses to the patients and make sure they understood them, instead of just diagnosing them and sending them on their way.

It takes certain qualities and skills to be a great physician assistant, and I believe I have those qualities and skills. I am patient, detail oriented, compassionate, and I work well both independently and as a team member. I also have great problem solving skills and I am very hard working. One quality that is very important is having great communication skills. This is one I have always struggled with, but working in the doctor's office has helped me significantly by having to communicate with patients all day.

Though I am not following the career path I thought I was going to be in high school, I am very much looking forward to continuing on in the physician assistant program. I am not completely sure what field of medicine I would like to work in yet, but I have a strong interest in sports medicine and orthopedics. I believe those interests stem from my athletic trainer in high school, and even though it is not exactly the same, I believe she had the greatest impact on me and helped me get to the position I am in today.

Commentary Essay 61

Your essay is earnest and genuine, two great qualities. It's good that you mention your difficulty with communicating, and that you've overcome it. If that's an issue when you get nervous (like in an interview setting), be sure to practice in advance with several people.

Your essay needs polishing, though. The opening is good, although it could be a little shorter. Read it again and take it to the bare necessities.

The second paragraph needs more work than the first, so I'm using that as an example of how your essay could be edited:

"Though I had never realized it, I have seen a PA since I was a baby. She always takes the time to talk to me, even if it is just for a cold or an ear infection. On the rare occasion that I see the doctor in the office, the visit always seems less personal. I believe that is one of the things that really drew me into pursuing this career – having the ability to develop patient-provider relationships."

The last sentence of that paragraph doesn't add anything to your essay, so it should come out.

You don't need to mention specific things you've learned in your job (those skills are secondary and not very critical in the scheme of things). That leaves you room to elaborate on work you've witnessed the PA do in more specific detail and why that appeals to you. You also give a list of your qualities. Do you use any of them in your work? If so, talk about that.

The last sentence of your conclusion could be a lot stronger. The focus shouldn't be on the athletic trainer, but on you. Sure, she inspired you, but you took that inspiration and turned it into a career goal.

By the way, physicians aren't someone PAs fall back on — they're the supervising medical professional. Be sure the way you word things properly conveys your understanding of the profession.

Essay 62

The sweat dripped down the faces of the Ghanaian villagers waiting in line to receive medical attention. Each villager had walked several miles of dirt roads and forest to get to our clinic. Each one had a look in their eye that was both fear of their health and hope that we could help them. It's this look that will forever be ingrained in my mind. We had been in the village for three days, partaking in ritualistic ceremonies, meeting with village leaders, visiting and explaining to the villagers about the clinic we were running. Our clinic consisted of dentists, doctors, OBGYN, phar-macy, and medical education presentations. The patients we saw ranged from elder to infant. I remember one patient; a little boy in the mother's arms had contracted malaria and needed medi-cal assistance. From the moment I saw the joy and relief sweep across the mother's face when we told her we could help her son, my passion to be involved in the medical field was reaffirmed. Running a week long clinic out of the village's 20' x 20' clay school and seeing over 500 patients from the local indigenous villages of Ghana made me realize that there is no greater honor than being able to provide someone medical care. I grew up hearing about the exemplary quality of healthcare in America. My mother came to America from South Korea when she was 24 to become a nurse in "the land of opportunity". I was constantly surrounded with stories from the hospital, but the things that stood out the most were the level of compassion and profession-alism that every medical professional seemed to bring to every patient. From a young age, there was no doubt in my mind that I wanted to be like my mom and the professionals she praised, and be involved in the field of medicine.

Though I had a goal, I lacked a specific path or direction not re-alizing the variety of careers available. By senior year I applied and was accepted in the Medical Program of the Peace Corps thinking that an experience caring for others abroad would help figure out a career path that suited me. While I waited to be de-ployed, I began work as an Operating Room Technician at The Ohio State Cancer Center. It was this position that first exposed me to Physicians Assistants.

Everything I learned about what is a physician assistant, peaked my interest. Being versatile in different fields mimicked how di-verse I was in campus organizations. Being able to bond with a variety of medical teams and patients resonated with my unique ability to relate to a lot of different types of people and connect and comfort them. An environment where you can put in your input, have independence, but still have some supervision for a different perspective is what I thrive in. That's what I love about teamwork, finding the balance of being confident in one's abilities but still humble enough to accept other people's opinions. My philosophy is a single person will not know everything, only working with others and immersing themselves in a team/interactions will they learn more then they were ever capable of. Every PA I shadowed embodied this, and with every shadowing experience my drive to become a PA increased.

My liberal arts education at Denison helped me become an excellent communicator and critical thinker – skills that will help me as a Physician's Assistant. My empathy, compassion and hardworking personality encouraged me to take on leadership positions on campus. Every group taught me something different about the world but also taught me something new about myself. Proudly being one of the only male members of Sexual Harassment And Rape Education (SHARE) I could reach out and provide comfort to students that had gone through traumatizing events. It was in this role that I learned that I could bring a personal form of compassion to care for others.

I learned a lot during my time at Denison, but I also made some mistakes. I did poorly on some big assignments in advanced courses, which resulted in lower grades. Despite that, the challenging courses I took helped me become a better communicator, take accountability for my actions and understand the importance of organization. With a career goal in mind, I am motivated to use those lessons more than ever, immersing myself into my work at the hospital taking advantage of being able to witness complex surgeries and interact with top-notch medical teams. My dedication to this profession is also exemplified by my willingness to take extra classes after graduation to meet the course requirements and boost my GPA.

I am proud of the journey I've had thus far. My trip to Ghana and my experience this past year working in a Cancer hospital has made me both excited and motivated to become a PA. I know that I will successfully use the knowledge acquired from the people around me, courses I've taken, and my compassionate nature, to become a great physician assistant and make a positive impact in every life I interact with.

Commentary Essay 62

You've done a great job on your essay. It starts with a compelling health care related situation, explains poor grades, and focuses on your recent experiences.

A couple very minor grammar things. Don't capitalize physician assistant. Same with cancer unless it's part of a name like The Ohio State Cancer Center." This portion of your third sentence, "Each one had a look in their eye" should read "All had a look in their eyes. . ." Quotes go outside of punctuation, "the land of opportunity". should be "the land of opportunity." Grammar errors can be fatal to an application according to the Admissions Directors I interviewed.

You have a few awkward sentences, such as this one: "Everything I learned about what is a physician assistant, peaked my interest," and "With a career goal in mind, I am motivated to use those lessons more than ever, immersing myself into my work at the hospital taking advantage of being able to witness complex surgeries and interact with top-notch medical teams." Break up that last sentence and use "in my work" instead of "into my work."

The sentence that begins with "I grew up . . ." should be the start of a new paragraph. You could shorten that paragraph, too, which will make the point but not belabor it. Here's how it could be edited:

My mother came to America from South Korea when she was 24 to become a nurse in "the land of opportunity." I constantly heard stories about the hospital, but the things that stood out were the compassion and professionalism that every medical professional brought to patients. From a young age, there was no doubt that I wanted to be like those professionals, involved in the field of medicine.

Look at your other paragraphs, too, and see where you can eliminate words to tighten things ups. Remember, your readers are seeing thousands of essays, and you want them to get your message quickly and efficiently.

Overall, though, I have little to complain about!

Essay 63

A surge of adrenaline rushes through my system as the words "CODE 99" hit me like icy water; I feel my heart immediately pound and I run. Being on the code team in the hospital fills me with immense euphoria and gratification. We are given the opportunity to provide immediate, lifesaving care to patients in critical condition. The environment is fast paced, and I appreciate working toward the same goal with people from different departments, with different skill sets. It is during these moments, I am reminded of the importance of teamwork and how strongly it appeals to me.

I discovered the significance of team based care in the physician assistant (PA) profession by shadowing various health care workers. Not only did I love the excitement and the intellectual challenges I observed while shadowing a PA, but also the collaborative work she did with the physician while retaining a level of autonomy. The relationship between the physician and the PA allowed the PA to be a true extension of the physician. I observed her not only as a second pair of skilled hands in the operating room, but also examining the patient before and after the surgery. She was involved in every aspect of the practice in concert with the physician.

The attraction to teamwork may be rooted in my love of competitive tennis. On the court, your doubles game is dependent on the harmony you share with your partner. To be successful, it is crucial to know your role and to be able to efficiently communicate with your partner while a point is live and in play. The same idea behind success applies in thriving PA physician relationships.

As a math major in college, my mind naturally falls into thinking about the world in terms of its fundamental units and analyzing the underlying patterns. I am drawn to the PA profession because I want to solve patients' illnesses. The various theorems, laws and postulates used to obtain a solution in mathematics are the different tests and procedures needed to determine a diagnosis in medicine. Once a potential diagnosis is reached, a second problem with new variables emerges; how to treat the illness. In the same way that I craved complex and difficult problems, I crave more medical training and knowledge to earn new responsibilities.

While in college, I had my first experience in patient interaction. I volunteered fulltime at a community health clinic in Suva, Fiji. The language barrier, a challenge that seemed difficult to overcome, proved to open up a new world of perception. For the first time, I could not rely on verbal communication, and I began to truly understand and develop empathy. For me, this emphasized the importance of trying to understand the world from the patient's perspective.

Although I underperformed during certain semesters in my undergraduate education, I am very proud to have rediscovered my focus and determination over these past years. As I have matured, I have become much better at time management and focusing on the task at hand. My patients demand it from me and I demand it from myself. Therefore, I refuse to let previous imperfect grades discourage me as I continue my education and involvement in health care. Recently, in addition to taking several science courses, I have received a CNA license and underwent training in phlebotomy and EKGs. Balancing my academic studies with the demands of a fulltime job over the last several years has ultimately heightened my ability to thrive in a graduate program at your institution.

My work and volunteer experiences have taught me the demands, thrills, and frustrations of being a health care provider. I have developed the ability to help people and the commitment to becoming a compassionate and responsible physician assistant. This profession is the best fit for my medical interests and career goals because it encompasses my passion for teamwork, knowledge, and impact. This is the path I have chosen, and I am committed to making the necessary sacrifices to achieve this goal.

Commentary Essay 63

This is an excellent start to your personal statement. You've covered a lot of territory and included key components that Admissions Directors look for in an essay. Your writing is very good — a big plus.

I'd recommend toning down the opening a bit. You don't want it to sound overdramatic (every Admissions person I interviewed said ditch the melodrama). Besides, you don't want to sound like you panic every time you hear code 99. It would be more effective to write something like this: "Adrenaline surges as I hear the words "CODE 99," and I run."

The second paragraph is excellent. I'm not sure you need the third, but if you have room, you can leave it in because it shows a deeper understanding of the importance of teamwork. When speaking of teamwork, though, don't focus exclusively on the physician. There are other team members, too. Remember, also, that being a PA is not only about teamwork. See if you can weave in other aspects of the job in more detail. You mention briefly that the PA examines the patient before and after, but relate that back to teamwork. Tie it to another aspect of the job.

There's no transition to the fourth paragraph, and I'm a little concerned that it makes you seem too distant from patient care and more interested in theoretical science and medicine. I know that's not true, but take a good look at that paragraph and see if you can't sound a bit more human when talking about how math relates to medicine. You could omit that paragraph entirely (it doesn't do much for the essay). I'd like to see you focus on your experiences with patients while volunteering and working. You say you developed empathy. Show us by letting us see you interact with patients. That's currently missing from your essay.

You did an excellent job of explaining less than stellar grades. You owned it, then showed how you won't let that stop you from pursuing a career as a PA.

With a bit of rewriting, you'll have a great essay.

Essay 64

Imagine living in a country where being without health insurance is practically a death sentence. I was born in Ukraine, a country where this is a reality. At the age of 3, I immigrated to the United States with my parents. After several years, my mother started attending a community college and eventually became an ultrasound technician. One thing that she spoke to me about almost every day was the quality of healthcare in America. Not only did we have groundbreaking medical research, innovative machines and diagnostic tests, and arguably the best medical education in the world, but we had caring medical professionals. These were individuals that would never leave someone to die due to their lack of ability to pay out-of-pocket medical expenses, as was relatively common in Ukraine. Listening to my mother speak so highly of medical professionals was what originally sparked my interest in healthcare. I wanted to have a career from which I could come home at the end of the day and know that I helped someone or changed a life. There was never any question that medicine was the path for me.

I started my undergraduate education on scholarship at The Ohio State University on a Pre Medicine track with the plan of becoming a doctor. At the time, I didn't realize how many careers there were in medicine outside of doctors and nurses. My first semester, I started volunteering at a hospital. It was while volunteering that I first came across physician assistants. While speaking with the receptionist one day, she asked me why I wanted to be a doctor. I told her about my love of medicine, my interest in various medical specialties and my desire to help people for a living. It was then that she mentioned physician assistants and how they do all of the things that I love about medicine but with a shorter education and more flexibility in switching fields. When I got home that day, I started researching the field and the more I learned, the more I felt like I had found my calling. I spent the rest of that semester deliberating whether medical school or PA school would be right for me.

Before I made my decision, I spent some time shadowing and that was what ultimately convinced me that I wanted to be a physician assistant. While shadowing a PA in orthopedics, I noticed how she seemed to have a knack for explaining things in layman's terms, something that the doctor on the unit didn't seem to have enough time for with over 30 patients per day. The PAs split the patients amongst themselves, leaving them with more time to provide patient care and a listening ear, not just medical expertise. The particular physician assistant that I shadowed took the time to explain the patient's condition to him, what they planned to do to fix it, showed him X-rays, and used a simple explanation for his condition. I could tell when we left the room just how grateful the patient was to have someone sit down and make sure all his questions were answered before leaving the room. It was after that shadowing experience that I dedicated my next three years of college to getting into PA school and every step I've taken since then was with the intention of becoming a physician assistant.

As I proceeded through my college education, I became involved with many extracurricular activities that were extremely stimulating for both my personal and professional development as a future healthcare provider. Although I was involved in many organizations, I was most influenced by my volunteer experiences, shadowing, and eventually my job as an Operating Room Technician. One volunteering opportunity that impacted my life was a service trip to Atlanta, GA through the organization BuckIServ, in which we worked in impoverished neighborhoods doing various tasks from tutoring to helping sort food at a food bank. The work that we did there did not necessarily pertain to healthcare, but I found the lessons and experiences gained from this trip to be very applicable to medicine. Working with the less fortunate taught me about the complicatedness of poverty. I began to realize that the side of healthcare that I had been seeing in the hospital was only one side of the story. An injection or drug could only do so much for a condition when a person isn't able to afford nutritional food, or understand the instructions the doctor provides due to lack of sufficient education. Sometimes an understanding of the person as a whole is more important for treating an illness than knowledge of a disease from a textbook. This realization has absolutely changed the way I view medicine and something I will always keep in mind when I am treating patients.

In the summer before my third year of college, I secured a job as an Operating Room Technician at the James Cancer Hospital. My job duties could be described as "anything and everything that needs to be done around the OR". I am in charge of making sure rooms are stocked between surgeries, getting equipment for the rooms during surgery, running cultures and specimens to labs, helping get patients into the operating room and prepared for surgery, and so much more. I truly feel like a valuable member of the healthcare team in providing care to patients and I swell with pride every time a patient wakes up from anesthesia in a panic and I am able to calm them and explain that we are taking care of them and actually see them relax. I am fortunate to have the opportunity to spend my free time at work watching complex surgeries and speaking to doctors and their physician assistants about the procedures they are performing. I have learned that every medical decision that is made takes into account many factors and that no two patient situations are the same and must be treated as such. I look forward to the day when I have the knowledge and expertise to make these decisions. It's a task that I embrace with open arms because the more time I spend immersed in medicine, the more excited I am to start my formal education as a physician assistant.

Commentary Essay 64

After learning about the dire consequences of the lack of medical care options in your birth country, and hearing your mother talk about healthcare in the U.S., I understand your desire to pursue a career in medicine. You've done a lot of work to get to the point of applying.

You did a great job of explaining why you decided to go the PA route as opposed to any other. You'd be surprised how many people never mention why they want to be a PA. The problem with your essay is that it will be hard for the Admissions folks to remember that because the essay is way too long (you're over 6,000 characters) and loses focus in all the unnecessary words.

Your opening for example, has too much information. I'm also not sure if the way the essay is formatted here is the way you've written it. If so, the first paragraph should be four separate paragraphs.

After editing, this is how the first two paragraphs of your essay could read:

"Imagine living in a country where being without health insurance is practically a death sentence. I was born in Ukraine, where this is a reality.

After my family immigrated to the United States, my mother became an ultrasound technician. One thing that she spoke to me about almost daily was the quality of healthcare in America. Listening to her sparked my interest in having a career from which I could come home at the end of the day and know that I helped someone or changed a life. There was never any question that medicine was the path for me."

Scrutinize every word and ask yourself, "Does this help the Admissions person reading my essay know me?" For example, no one will care that a receptionist mentioned PAs to you. That's the kind of thing I'm talking about. In fact, you could delete most of that paragraph.

Once you cut away all the fat, you'll be left with an excellent essay.

Essay 65

Topless and shaking with tears in her eyes, she stopped me. "Thank you," she said, and smiled. I stood there alone with her, swallowing the tears that had formed in my own eyes and nodded, smiling back. This was the first time I had ever been in a situation like this and soon found out it wouldn't be the last. Dr. Carter had left the room to speak with Laura's* breast surgeon. She had been diagnosed with an invasive ductal carcinoma in her right breast and surgery was scheduled for the following week. She was here to discuss the possibility of reconstruction, mostly because she was told to come. Laura was scared and overwhelmed; she didn't know what steps to take, or what lie ahead. At the end of the hour we spent together, she told me that for the first time since her diagnosis, which had been given to her quite impersonally over the phone, she felt like she was in good hands. As I stood there with Laura, who was still half-dressed, she began laughing at herself for forgetting her decency. Laura got dressed as I walked her through the next few days, going through a rough timeline of the next couple of months, including potential chemotherapy, radiation, and the subsequent visits we would have with her for reconstruction.

In my time working for Dr. Carter, a Plastic and Reconstructive Surgeon in Washington, D.C., I've had the pleasure of working with countless patients like Laura, each with his or her own story and reason for being in Dr. Carter's office. Working in this office, I have learned that exemplary patient care relies on a dedication to seeing each patient as an individual while taking the time to not only treat their ailments, but to provide comprehensive care. Before Laura left that day, I walked her downstairs and made her an appointment with an oncologist, introduced her to the staff in the oncology suite, and made sure she knew exactly where she was going and how to prepare for her surgery that coming week.

Over the past year and a half, my responsibilities at Dr. Carter's office have grown to encompass more than just day to day patient care. I am personally responsible for seeing my patients through, from the preop preparation to postop care and discharge, and anything that may occur in between. As a liaison between Dr. Carter and her patients, I learned the importance of developing a high degree of trust between myself and the patients I work with, as well as with the various medical professionals I coordinate care with on a daily basis. My academic background, patient care experience, and volunteer services have all helped to thoroughly prepare me for the duties and responsibilities a Physician's Assistant often faces. The role I have as a medical assistant is something I have greatly enjoyed doing. The connections I was fortunate to have had with Laura as well as those with countless other patients are experiences I look forward to cultivating for the rest of my life. Developing the next stages in my career towards becoming a Physician's Assistant is something I look forward to every day, and I would be honored to be a part of your program. Thank you for your time and consideration.

*Patient name has been changed for privacy.

Commentary Essay 65

This is very well done as far as it goes. I love that you open with Laura's story. (By the way, name her in the first sentence: "Topless and shaking with tears in her eyes, Laura stopped me" and then write what she stopped you from — continuing your explanation of the timeline for her treatment plan, for example. The sentence doesn't make sense as it's written now). There's a lot of great info about how you've developed your skills through your work experiences. Dr. Carter's patients are lucky!

What's really missing from your essay is why you want to be a PA. You point out (very well, I might add) that your job has prepared you for assuming responsibilities of a PA, but that's as far as it goes. "Why the PA profession?" This is something that every Admissions Director and faculty member I spoke with said was crucial to the essay. Have you shadowed or worked with a PA? If so, what about those experiences do you relate to? What aspects of the job appeal to you? Or if you haven't, you'll need to tell how you know about the profession and what led you in that direction.

You may need to cut some of what you've written to fit that in. It won't be hard if you take a close look at your essay. There are words here and there you can delete. For example, you could delete this sentence and it would never be missed: "The role I have as a medical assistant is something I have greatly enjoyed doing." We get that from your essay.

Your essay has good bones. Now it needs to be fleshed out.

Essay 66

The pavement flies by as one big smooth charcoal blur. I grip my handle bars as if they are my life support. Pedaling nonstop as my heart pounds and adrenaline pumps through my body I pedal faster and faster. Neck to neck with my opponent, my legs and chest burn with pain as I push myself harder than I think is possible. Excitement, stress and determination all build up in me as I sprint for the finish. Six feet, four feet, two feet and I cross the finish line inches behind my opponent. Mustering up the courage, I congratulate the winner and she tells me that this was her first win after several years of racing. Not only did she deserve it, I was ecstatic knowing it was my first race ever as a collegiate road cyclist and I finished in the top three. When I think about why I put myself through the intense pain and hard work that it takes to be a competitive cyclist, I am reminded that it is determination that fuels the desires of my heart. My desire to become a physician assistant (PA) comes from the same place.

The mind and the heart work differently, both realistically and figuratively, but I know it is possible to have the desires of the heart naturally align to the logic of the mind. I am an example of this. My heart longs to show compassion and empathy to others while my mind needs to be stimulated scientifically and analytically. After researching, shadowing and working in the medical field I have found that a career as a physician assistant satisfies the desires of my heart and is best suited to my skills and personality.

Having majored in health studies within the public health education discipline, I took many classes that focused on community health and health disparities. I understand that the health of an individual involves more than just that person, it involves the whole community. It is my desire to combine my knowledge of both fields to improve the health of a whole community by educating and empowering individuals. Additionally, I enjoy working and collaborating as a team while still having autonomy to make important decisions. I saw this first hand when I shadowed a PA. I don't like the idea of being confined to just one area of medicine. I want the option of changing specialties to expand my knowledge of the human body without having to go through another residency program, which is why I decided not to become a doctor.

Deep down I have always felt a strong inkling to want to make a difference in the lives of the people I encounter. Working as a certified nursing assistant is one way I have been able to do that. As one of the younger nursing aids in my facility, I am able to use my youthful energy and good humor to brighten my patient's day. It is quite extraordinary to see how much a small gesture like a smile can greatly impact someone's life. Working as a nursing assistant has been the most challenging work I have ever done; I truly love it, but I need to utilize my analytical ways of thinking and creative methods to solving problems to be fulfilled in a career. I need to be more involved in the diagnostics and treatment of patients, beyond the nursing modality.

Cycling and a career in medicine share several similarities. Long hours spent conditioning and preparing yourself for the road ahead. Having a plan of attack to overcome any obstacle is vital to success because even the most athletic riders and prominent medical professionals risk losing without a strategy. Lastly, having a team that is supportive and communicates well positively affects the outcome of any obstacle. The intensity of feelings that draw me into my bike saddle every day, that push me beyond my physical limit originate because I am determined. The road ahead may be stressful and even painful at times, but I am determined to finish, even if it's second best.

Commentary Essay 66

Good job on the essay. It's upbeat, even exuberant. The second paragraph is stellar. And you did a good job of saying what you like about being a PA. Of course, I still have some suggestions. A minor one — everyone knows PA stands for physician assistant, so you don't need to explain it.

I suggest you shorten the first paragraph. It's descriptive, but you could make your point in less words. I'd like to see that ability to describe focused on a PA or CNA related patient instead. Take a few sentences to let the reader see you really get what being a PA is about.

This is how I'd edit the first sentence:

The pavement flies by and I grip my bicycle handle bars as if they are my life support. Pedaling nonstop as my heart pounds and adrenaline pumps, I'm neck to neck with my opponent. My legs and chest burn as I push myself harder than I think is possible. Excitement, stress and determination all build as I sprint for the finish. I cross the finish line inches behind my opponent. It was my first race as a collegiate road cyclist and I finished in the top three. When I think about why I put myself through the hard work to be a competitive cyclist, I am reminded that determination fuels the desires of my heart. My desire to become a physician assistant comes from the same place.

I'd probably leave out that you don't want to be confined to one area of medicine, and end the next sentence at "body." It tells the readers what they need to know framed in a positive, not negative way.

The word "inkling" doesn't work. Use something stronger, like interest or desire. You'll need to rewrite that sentence.

And whatever you do, take out the last phrase of the conclusion. You don't want anyone to think you're satisfied with or only worthy of second best.

Essay 67

There is nothing I love better than a good challenge. I used to be a sprinter on the track team in high school. My favorite events were the short races that were all about pure speed until I discovered hurdling and I immediately fell in love. There is a quote that says "Hurdlers are sprinters with a problem. They're not satisfied just to sprint. Anybody can sprint...Not everybody can run hurdles. There's an extra dimension involved. Hurdlers...are of a persuasion that just needs an extra dimension." It was exactly that extra dimension that pulled me in and quickly transformed me from a sprinter into a hurdler. Before I knew it I was training for a pentathlon, and I had become both mentally and physically stronger as a result.

My involvement in emergency medicine followed a similar progression. I joined URI's volunteer ambulance corps as a recruit and loved it so much that I decided to earn my EMT license. In time I became a Field Training Officer and a Corporal in order to share my knowledge and serve as a role model to my peers. Once I became comfortable as a care provider, I decided to go the extra mile and earn my EMT Cardiac license to become an advanced life support provider. Many people asked me why I was bothering. "Won't you only learn a few more skills?" or "Aren't you busy enough as it is?" For me the answer was simple. I knew I had what it took to reach the next level, and I was not going to let the opportunity to expand upon my knowledge pass me by.

The class was an hour drive twice a week and began just before final exams. I was the only woman in a class of male firefighters, most of whom were much older than me. I had to work hard to keep up with my workload and be taken seriously by my classmates. But I loved what I was doing and could not have been prouder to finally earn my license. When you put your heart and soul into what you are passionate about, going the extra mile feels more like a personal victory lap. It is a celebration of refusing to settle for the minimum and always striving to reach your fullest potential. That is one of the best feelings in the world.

Similar to the way track strengthened me physically and mentally, my experience in EMS has strengthened my character in ways I never imagined. I have gained more confidence in myself than I never knew I could possess, and acquired the skills to become an effective leader and teacher to my peers. I have learned how to take charge of difficult situations and be the calm in the storm during the worst times in people's lives. In addition, I have increased my capacity for compassion. The ability to connect with patients on a personal level and communicate that you are there for them is often just as important as high-quality medicine. This point was driven home for me one night in the emergency room. An older man was lying in bed while his wife hovered nervously around him. As a nurse went in to check on him, he suddenly became unresponsive. The room became a flurry of activity and I ran over, eager to help save this man's life. Instead I found myself walking over to the man's panicked wife and gently steering her out of the room. I calmly explained that the ER team was doing everything they could and that I would sit with her the entire time. In the end her husband was resuscitated and admitted to the hospital. Before she followed him upstairs she walked over to me and grabbed my hand. She looked at me with tears in her eyes and simply whispered, "Thank you". Sometimes going the extra mile is as simple as letting someone know they are not alone.

I love every minute that I spend in the back of an ambulance, but I know I could not be content with doing this job for the rest of my life. I used to think that my next step would be medical school, but the more I learned about physician assistants the more I knew that it was right for me. Good medicine is never a one man show and the PA profession offers a great opportunity to work as a team player. It offers the flexibility to make lateral moves and experience different specialties, as well as delve into the realm of public health at the same time. I was ecstatic when I realized that a handful of programs across the country offered a dual degree option for PA and Master of Public Health. Some people settle for one aspect of medicine but I feel compelled to meet the challenge of helping bridge the clinical and humanistic sides of medicine. I believe that becoming a PA would put me in the perfect position to do just that. I have been fortunate enough to shadow several remarkable PAs, and have observed the same attitude with each one. These people are not in it for glory, but for the love of practicing medicine. That is the type of healthcare provider that I want to be and I know PA school is the way to get there. The road will not be easy and there will be many times when going the extra mile will feel like a marathon, but I am confident that I am up to the challenge.

Commentary Essay 67

This is quite well done. I suspect you've spent a lot of time polishing it, and your efforts have paid off.

I just have a few suggestions. First shorten the quote (it's awkward as written) and attribute it properly. You could do this: Denny Moyer said, "Hurdlers are sprinters with a problem. They're not satisfied just to sprint . . . they are of a persuasion that just needs an extra dimension."

You could eliminate this sentence: "When you put your heart and soul into what you are passionate about, going the extra mile feels more like a personal victory lap." The next sentence says the same thing. Pick one or the other. Personally, I think the second is stronger.

Take out this: "Some people settle for one aspect of medicine but." It sounds like you're putting others down, which I know is not your intention. You don't need it, anyway.

If you read your essay with a very critical eye, you'll find other places to take out a few words here and there and still make your important points. It will just make it easier for the reader, who has to slog through 1,000-2,000 essays.

Other than that, I think you're in great shape.

Essay 68

Most would say that first impressions leave a permanent mark. However, I believe in last impressions.

For example, I don't recall my first thoughts when I had a herpes outbreak at twelve years old. It hurt to laugh or grin, although I had no reason to from the ridicule I endured. Weary of the derision, I read to escape and learned that HSV1 was transmittable by sharing utensils. Having the virus became less of a social stigma for me – I found comfort in that. The scabs healed and the kids targeted their next prey but my insatiable curiosity remained. As I explored why the way things were, I began to see the world differently. Fading horizons came from the earth's spin, hinting at invisible rays. A spectrum of wavelengths colored early dawns and late dusks, hemming the day in its embrace. The relatively little I knew about the functions of the body made everyone a breathing work of art. I've grown to admire every aspect of the universe in a language that is universal.

My penchant in finding scientific truths persisted within my academic studies through research. However, I longed for clinical interactions. Seeking opportunities, I immersed myself in collaborative healthcare orientated organizations that led me to countless of career pathways. I initially felt overwhelmed in an unfamiliar setting but I adapted my skills in studying and time management. As I explored the gamut of healthcare professions, being a PA grew more enticing each time. From working in dermatology to researching cardiology, I revel in subjects I've engrossed myself in. The flexibility among the broad range of specialties was ideal to comply accordingly with the demand from communities. This unique facet of the profession offers infinite ways to employ analytical aspects of medicine while supporting a rewarding lifestyle.

Ergo, I shadowed Mr. Imbus. Welcoming my inquisitive nature, he explained the arduous nature of being a Neurology PA and showed how to do it well. He confidently evaluated his patients and reviewed their treatments with charisma. His dedication exhibited the quality care I yearned to emulate in the healthcare field. At my last session, he explained why he decided against being a doctor like his father: "Growing up, my dad missed one too many of my baseball games. I didn't want that for my kids." The idea that time is a merciless hourglass, with sand seeping to the inevitable, resonated with me. His hourglass had ample sand to be with his family longer and to heal patients sooner.

Our final encounter made me ponder how I wanted to make the most out of my time. I embarked on a summer medical trip to Nicaragua after a year of saving up. The line was endless at the makeshift clinics, but most were seizing the only chance they had to receive medical care. It was a luxury that depended on students and healthcare providers harmonizing together efficiently, a riveting process that I was excited to engage in. Mia, a patient, was uncomfortable at first. But it was amazing how smiling and body language transcended cultural barriers. Tensions dwindled, the creases of her sun kissed skin waved around her eyes as she smiled. Her back relaxed with each breath undulating along the stethoscope. Placating the mistrust she harbored reaffirmed my aspirations. After studying science academia for so long, performing its practical applications was vitalizing. We treated the symptoms before. Now, we treated the person. There was a deep fulfillment none like it.

From their trials, the patients emerged as stronger people. But they came from a vast demographic suffering from inaccessible healthcare, bolstering my urgency to aid the underprivileged like Mia. Hovels and cardboard boxes acted more as shelters than homes. Lack of education and unsanitary conditions made the few resources that villages had often tainted. Our duty was not just to deter death but to improve the quality of life too. The sooner patients are seen, the sooner they'd be relieved of their suffering at the very least.

I expected to change lives by giving courage to the discouraged. But in the end, the patients made the trip life changing for me as well. Despite their hardships, they made the best of their situation with jokes and laughter. When I get dismayed, I'm reminded of their resilience. My desire to help the afflicted had never wavered; it had only been fortified. As Mia told me, boiling water softens the potato and hardens the egg — it's what one's made of, not of one's circumstances. Every great challenge comes with a great opportunity for growth. I can only hope that this outlook will have a reassuring effect on those around me, especially my patients.

I believe in making last impressions. Being a PA is my way of doing so. This decision wasn't a single pivotal moment, but rather a myriad of personal and academic experiences accruing over time. To this day, I reminiscence over the impact people have left on me. Now, I'm determined to leave a positive impact on others.

Commentary Essay 68

Great job on the theme for your essay, and on bringing it full circle. I love Mia's saying about boiling water. That's priceless.

In fact, the essay is quite well done except for one thing — the over the top adjectives. The flowery, melodramatic writing is distracting and takes away from the impact that recounting your experiences could have. Unfortunately, it's found throughout.

Take these sentences for example: "Fading horizons came from the earth's spin, hinting at invisible rays. A spectrum of wavelengths colored early dawns and late dusks, hemming the day in its embrace. The relatively little I knew about the functions of the body made everyone a breathing work of art. I've grown to admire every aspect of the universe in a language that is universal." They're pretty, but what do they tell the reader about you? How will they help an Admissions Director determine that you might be a great PA?

Here are other examples: "The idea that time is a merciless hourglass, with sand seeping to the inevitable, resonated with me," "creases of her sun-kissed skin waved around her eyes," each breath undulating along the stethoscope," "harmonizing together efficiently, a riveting process," "reviewed their treatments with charisma." I can't visualize how creases wave around eyes or how you review treatments with charisma. The problem is that the writing made me stop and think about it.

The goal of the personal statement is to catch your reader's eye. Flowery language is not the way to do it. Go through your essay and write the second through fourth paragraphs like the last two paragraphs (well, except for "bolstering my urgency"). Then you'll have a winner.

Essay 69

I was married a little longer than a year when my world collapsed and separated into "before and after". Our bright future together, dreams and new beginnings shot down in a minute I woke up to my husband screaming with an inhuman voice. He never talked about his past, but I realized it was something extremely dark in his memories. A couple nights later he woke up screaming in terror again. From that, the amplitude of his nightmares started to grow bigger and became more violent. Just in a few weeks he became his own shadow with blackened eyes, poor posture, skinnier than ever. Seeking answers, I read an article about psychiatric diseases. The symptoms conclusively confirmed that my husband was suffering from traumatic events that led to severe posttraumatic stress disorder. It took six months to convince him to accept the help. These six months I spent researching cases, treatments, and supporting groups. These six months changed my perception of the world, and, despite my prior experience and academic choices, I realized that I wanted to help people when they were sick.

I changed my major to pre-nursing and soon got accepted into the nursing school. The first year in the nursing program I recognized that nursing scope of practice would not be enough for what I wanted to accomplish: I needed independence; I needed an extensive and in depth training; I wanted to practice medicine on a team and under supervision; I wanted to not only examine patients but also be able to diagnose and provide treatment. With that in mind, I began researching my options until I found the Physician Assistant profession. The more I learned about the profession, the more amazed I became of the impact that could be done to the patient's life by a PA. I continued my research of the profession and available programs. That helped me create the list of prerequisite classes I needed to complete to become a competitive applicant. I proceeded with nursing education, while taking prerequisite classes and working. In May 2014, I graduated with an Associate Degree in Nursing, and immediately transitioned to Bachelor Degree in Nursing. Also, I was offered a job as a Registered Nurse in a local hospital. Last spring semester I was enrolled in three colleges, completing 22 credit hours. Working the night shifts in a busy step down unit I've met many clinicians: physicians, nurse practitioners and PAs. I've witnessed how different PAs interacted with nurses and physicians. I was amazed with the level of the comprehension, commitment, and patience PAs expressed towards patients and their families. Often, they would encourage patients to ask questions, and would provide extremely knowledgeable and easy to understand recommendations. From nurse's prospective PAs were the best clinicians to get instructions from: orders were clear, logical and thorough.

One of our PA who knew that I'm getting ready to apply for PA school told me: "Follow your dream and study hard". From a very young age, I knew exactly what "follow your dreams" really means. When I was four my mother, the piano teacher, had a heated discussion with my dad, the ballet dancer, if I should become a pianist. Every day since that conversation I was entitled to hours of practice behind my instrument. It started from four hours and ended at ten hours a day, every day, no days off, sick or vacation time. "I have no life," I thought, when I was fourteen. Now, I believe that all these days of practice built the stamina of my character. By the age of sixteen, I thrice performed with symphonic orchestra and won dozens of competitions. At eighteen, I have torn connective tissue in my hand while practicing, and became permanently incapable of performing at the professional level. I changed the venue of my talents and started education in advertising. The first year in, I became a class representative, and started working on thesis. By the third year, I had four publications, visited five conferences as a speaker, and got a job at the best advertising agency in the area. It was an exciting time when I had to manage my school, work and social life. The advertising agency I worked for was unfortunate to contract the political leader who became a strong opponent to the political frontrunner of the current (country's name) regime. The conflict of interest was established, and I and a few of my colleagues, who fought for its political beliefs, were recommended to leave the country. I left everything behind and started over.

Looking back at my life experiences, I truly believe that I needed to go through those difficulties to become a solid person. My husband's illness introduced me to the wonderful world of medicine. Every day I'm thankful for the progress we both made. He recovered with the help of his service animal, and I found my dream. There is no other answer to the question "Whom you want to become?". For me, it is the only answer. I want to become the Physician Assistant.

Commentary Essay 69

You've had a lot of life experience, all of which has made you the person you are now. But you don't need to include it all in your essay, and especially not in such detail. The result is that your essay is disorganized and hard to follow.

Instead of starting with your husband's illness, why not start with being forced to leave your country and start over? You'll need to shorten your description of the events, in fact, shorten it to two sentences. The move was hard, but made you a stronger person. Then it gives you the opportunity to transition to your husband's illness.

Leave out the part about the piano altogether. It's from your childhood and not as relevant as your current experiences.

You've got grammatical errors, such as putting a period after a quotation mark instead of before and mixing up your tenses. I suspect English may not be your first language and that has its own special set of challenges. For example, sayings, like your husband became his own shadow should be "he became a shadow of himself."

Here's how you could edit the paragraph about your husband:

I was married a little longer than a year when my world collapsed and separated into "before and after." Our bright future and dreams were shot down the minute I woke up to my husband screaming. The nightmares continued, and in just in a few weeks he became a shadow of himself. Seeking answers, I read about psychiatric diseases and realized my husband was suffering severe post-traumatic stress disorder. It took six months to convince him to accept help. Those six months changed my perception of the world, and, despite my prior experience and academic choices, I realized that I wanted to help people when they were sick."

By eliminating some of the details I've mentioned, you could expand on why you want to be a PA and how your skills will help make you a good one.

Have several people read your essay to make sure you've got your grammar right and that it's properly organized.

Essay 70

There are few people in life that, when you first encounter them, you know will somehow set you upon a whole new path; they will change the very fabric of who you are. The story of why I want to be a Physician Assistant, and my path to get to this essay, starts with Coach Whit – my sprint coach at Gettysburg College. An imposing figure, he exemplified and preached all of the principles he learned from his years in the Marine Corps – dedication, discipline, and character. Coach Whit was the first person to ever sit me down, look me in the eye, and say, "You have greatness. You just need to believe and work hard with unyielding passion." Belief is an intensely powerful thing and that belief in me, that support he carried for me, still pushes me to this day.

And, much like people, there are a precious few days in life that will begin a marvelous cascade of events that will change...well, everything. It was a Spring day on the track at Gettysburg College that was marked by two major incidents. First, the announcement that Coach Whit had lost his yearlong battle with cancer. Second, during practice that followed, I felt a pop in my leg that would sideline me for the rest of the season and then some. That one injury changed the entire path of my career.

I spent the next six months seeing specialist after specialist to diagnose the injury – athletic trainers, surgeons, and orthopedic and family doctors. While Coach Whit believed I would be something great, my own belief began to wane as the pain just walking to class was unbearable as these medical professionals told me "nothing was wrong." Finally, a physician who introduced himself as Jason sat down, and, for the first time, looked beyond the tests and actually seemed to listen to me. He explained the tests were negative but there is more to medicine than just testing. In a long shot move, he referred me out to a specialist in Milwaukee who diagnosed me with two hernias. Upon surgery, they found a third. This sanity saving conversation was not with a physician at all, however. In my naivety for the profession at the time, I never realized it was with a Physician Assistant.

Shortly after my recovery, I talked to a college advisor about becoming a PA who told me that I was too far behind in my science coursework; my grades were not high enough; I did not have enough experience nor did I have enough time even if I tried to catch up. I was too late and I should choose a different path. While I did not fully heed that advice, I also did not fully pursue this field because of that conversation. This resulted in a confused collegiate career that underwhelmed academically as I fought to find my way to help people the same way Coach Whit and Jason helped me. In my time after graduating, I have worked hard to show that I have the academic ability to thrive in PA school. Unfortunately, back then, I graduated more lost and further from my dream job than I thought possible.

However, two months into a job at Merrill Lynch postgraduation, I was offered an opportunity to go return and coach track and field. Ultimately, I knew it was a chance to pursue the prerequisites necessary to go to Physician Assistant school. A few days later, I left and started on a remarkable, difficult journey with nothing more than a dream, a chip on my shoulder, and a car full of clothes.

These past five years have forged me into a man of character, belief, dedication, and passion. I have been fighting to prove that, beyond all doubt, I can handle the academics, stress, challenge, and all of the rigors the programs present. I did not grow up wanting to be a Physician Assistant. I did not even enter college knowing what a Physician Assistant was. This is a career I discovered, fell in love with, chose amongst many others, sacrificed for, and fought for above all else.

And, in this journey, I have had to make great sacrifices that have forged me into a capable and mature student and professional. Although difficult to admit, I have been homeless twice; I have worked well over forty hours a week while going to school full time, earning nearly a 4.0 in sixteen courses; I have missed far more holidays with my family than I have made; I have felt the sting of a patient dying; the power of a tearful thank you from the scared and the sick. I have endured the swing shifts and the sleepless days and nights while working in the ER; the failure and repeat rejection; and have been blessed with the support and inspiration of remarkable clinicians, patients, and loved ones.

My path has not been an easy one. There were those mornings that I would wake up and ask myself, "Is this worth it? Is this something I really want to do?" The answer has unequivocally been "yes." On those days, I roll out of bed and smile, knowing I am one step closer to my dream and my goal. I keep what I learned from Coach Whit close: Believe – there is greatness inside of you.

Commentary Essay 70

Before I forget, physician assistant is not capitalized.

That aside, you've had quite a journey to get to this point. Congratulations on your perseverance through incredible adversity. It demonstrates your commitment and character.

You really need to shorten every paragraph. When I interviewed Admissions Directors and faculty, they all said personal experiences were okay as a way to open your essay, but they shouldn't dominate it. Make the second and third paragraphs into one paragraph a couple sentences long. The main point is you were injured and it was the PA who took the time to figure out what was wrong.

When you cut all the extra words, you'll have the opportunity to explain why you want to be a PA, what interests you about the profession and what you'll have to offer as a PA. You haven't done that in your essay. You obviously work in healthcare (doing what I can't tell). Expand on those experiences and how they've reinforced your desire to be a PA.

Here's an example of how you could edit the first paragraph:

"The story of why I want to be a physician assistant, and my path to this essay, starts with Coach Whit – my sprint coach at Gettysburg College. An imposing figure, he exemplified the principles he learned in the Marine Corps – dedication, discipline, and character. He was the first person to look me in the eye, and say, "You have greatness. You just need to believe and work hard with unyielding passion." His belief in me pushes me to this day."

Your conclusion is good. The tie back to Coach Whit brings you full circle.

Essay 71

"CORPSMAN UP". My first medical experience in a combat zone, I treated a Third Country National who had received shrapnel wound to his calf from a 50 caliber Machine Gun. His calf was almost completely blown out. Adrenaline started pumping and I started freaking out on the inside, my brain racing a "proverbial 100 miles an hour". All I could do was stop and force myself to take a deep breath. At that point in my career I had not had any experience with severe injuries, let alone combat injuries. However, what little training I had received kicked in and I was able to do what I needed to do to treat the casualty. After I turned him over to the combat hospital I walked outside and just started shaking. The adrenaline was finally leaving me. Looking back on that moment I was scared and excited all at once. The one thing I remember about afterwards, I went and asked the medical officers what I did wrong, what could I have done better. The tourniquet wasn't on tight enough, I didn't give him a proper turnover, but he did tell me what I did right, "you stayed calm".

Fast forward to 2013, laying in my rack in the Republic of Georgia, when entered a Georgian Soldier telling me to hurry there is a person that has been injured. I race to the site of the injury, all the while my mind a blur, ticking off my mental checklist. Upon arriving on scene, the area was in complete chaos. The Georgian medics were racing around trying to treat the patient. Calmly I intervened and quickly evaluated the patient, he was having a heart attack. Without any hesitation I proceeded to deliver CPR and calling for an immediate medevac. Once the AED was delivered, I began delivering "shocks". Helicopter lands and we are loaded, all the while I am still doing CPR and still utilizing the

AED. His airway was starting to close and the air wasn't being delivered properly. So I did something for the first time in my career, I inserted an Endotracheal tube. Having only inserted them into live animals, I didn't let my lack of experience stop me. First attempt was as you would expect, a jumbled mess. The second attempt I took a calm relaxing breath and I successfully got it in. For 45 minutes I performed CPR and defibrillated him, all the while staying calm. When we landed, I did once last vital sign check, no pulse, no breath signs. I assumed he had passed on. Once I turned over the patient, something didn't happen...I didn't shake, there was no adrenaline rush, just a calmness. Fortunately for the patient, he did survive, thanks in part to my actions. Two weeks later when I talked to an American military medical officer, I briefed them on what had occurred. I asked for suggestions on ways I could improve, I asked about things I did wrong, asking for training materials that I could learn from for the future.

The take away from these two experiences...I improved. From day one, I have been training and still train to this day. If I mess up, I figure out a way to not do it again. If it was done sloppy, I learn ways to improve my abilities. Becoming a Physician Assistant is an example of this. It is just another step in learning the art of medicine and improving my abilities. I am not the best, nor will I ever be the best, but the training and experience I learn from being a PA will go a long way towards making me be better at my job...being there for my patients when they need me the most. For me, my military experiences and training as a Hospital Corpsman have been the most of what I hope for in my medical career. As I continue in the Navy, I will decrease my patient interactions until finally I will not have anymore. PA is the next logical step, allowing me to continue doing what I love, patient care. From comforting a patient during a time of mourning, to getting the "Thank you very much" line from a patient you helped, to the bright smiles and hugs from patients. To those somber moments when you have to tell a patient that a "loved one" has passed on. These are moments that will live with me for the rest of my days. Being there for the patient is one of the greatest experiences and with your acceptance, I will be able to continue these experiences.

Commentary Essay 71

You've been able to do what few writers ever accomplish — telling a hot story cold. By that I mean, it's a straight forward telling of something horrific without the melodrama that usually accompanies it. Excellent work.

I recommend shortening what you've written about the experiences so you have room to write about why you want to become a PA. As I've said to others, Admissions Directors and faculty need to know that you understand what the profession involves and why it's right for you. I'm not sure you even need the second example. It makes the same point — you stayed calm and learned from your experiences.

You clearly have the capability of writing excellent descriptions. If you haven't shadowed a PA or worked with someone in the profession, then analogize from your experiences to show you understand what it takes to do the job.

Please don't be self-effacing. You want to come from a position of strength, not weakness.

For example, I would delete almost this entire part of the paragraph: "If I mess up, I figure out a way to not do it again. If it was done sloppy, I learn ways to improve my abilities. Becoming a Physician Assistant is an example of this. It is just another step in learning the art of medicine and improving my abilities. I am not the best, nor will I ever be the best, but the training and experience I learn from being a PA will go a long ways towards making me be better at my job...being there for my patients when they need me the most."

I might modify the first two sentences to read like this: "If I make mistakes, I learn ways to improve my abilities." Why specifically will being a PA go a long way toward making you better at a job or improve your skills? From the essay, I can't tell. You could be a nurse and improve your skills or be better at your job. You could be a doctor and do the same. Everything has to be PA specific.

Here's how I would edit your first paragraph (Notice that the period goes before the quote and it's afterward, not afterwards. I don't believe machine gun would be capitalized unless it's a brand. Is Third Country National a title? If not, don't capitalize the words. If he was a soldier, just say soldier, or a civilian, just say that):

"CORPSMAN UP." My first medical experience in a combat zone, I treated a Third Country National who had received shrapnel wound to his calf from a 50 caliber machine gun. His calf was almost completely blown out. Adrenaline started pumping and my brain was racing a 100 miles an hour. At that point in my career I had not had any experience with severe injuries, let alone combat injuries. However, what little training I had received kicked in and I was able to do what I needed to do. After I turned him over to the combat hospital I just started shaking. Looking back on that moment I was scared and excited all at once. Afterward, I went and asked the medical officer what could I have done better. The tourniquet wasn't tight enough, I learned. But he also told me what I had done right — I had stayed calm.

If you wrote, "The next time, I tied the tourniquet tight," it could be the last line of your paragraph. Then you can eliminate the second example altogether, which will give you space to write about the things I've mentioned.

Essay 72

"Whatever your heart desires, mine desires for you." This note was printed on the inside of a Valentine's Day card I received from an elderly patient during my second year as Certified Nursing Assistant (CNA). I cared for this patient nearly every morning and every evening for the first two years of my college career. At this point in my education I was working on my degree in International Studies. The patient that gave me this card knew the degree I was pursuing and knew the underlying passion driving this pursuit was a desire to help the underserved throughout the world. However, he also saw a passion within me that I had discarded during my high school years. He saw my eyes light up as he described his medical conditions and as I relayed medical research I had been reading in my spare time. I had told him that my plan all along was to go into medicine I grew up wanting to be a surgeon. However, in high school, I had decided that I would rather travel the world and help the populace on a larger scale and that pushed me to go into International Studies. One evening, I was telling this patient that I wasn't sure the International Studies field was going to be right for me. He took my hand and said "Sarah, I need you to become a doctor so you can take care of me and people like me."

Impassioned by these words, I used the following semester spent in Uganda to explore my deferred interest in medicine. I spent the later half of the semester in a hospital outside of Kampala with the intent of doing research on World Health Organization standards of care. I found myself so enthralled by the care being provided, by the procedures being done, I often forgot about my research and just reveled in the intricacies of caring for the human body. I learned that caring for the human body was the most basic way that an undeserved populace can be helped. These months spent in the surgical suites, outpatient clinics and medical wards allowed my two previously conflicting passions to be reconciled into one inextinguishable desire to learn about the human body and use that knowledge to help both at home and abroad.

Upon returning home, I wrapped up my degree in International Studies a year early in order to work full time and take medical prerequisites. It was during this time that I experimented with online coursework and decided that I could not learn through this medium. While I was still making a passable grade in my online Cellular Biology course, I decided to withdraw because I wasn't satisfied with the knowledge I was gaining. I was frustrated by not having a forum for discussion and information exchange through questions. I am "that student" in class that asks countless questions. I am a self-motivated learner; my desire to learn is driven by a deep seated curiosity. For the first time in my academic career, I knew that the information I was responsible for learning could one day be put to a real life application in the context of treating a patient. I took, and still take, this responsibility seriously and decided that on campus courses would better satiate my curiosity and desire to learn.

I began taking my prerequisites without knowing exactly where I wanted to go in the medical field. Shortly after graduation, I was fortunate enough to get a position as a Clinical Allergy Specialist working in a primary care office. I had volunteered in mental health, shadowed a pulmonologist, volunteered in public health, worked with the geriatric population in nursing homes and the female population in the OB/GYN clinic in Uganda, but I had never been exposed to the day in, day out consistent care provided by a primary care physician. I was worried that this exposure would dampen my interest in a career in medicine. It didn't. Rather, I was exhilarated each day when I was able to put the knowledge I was gaining in my prerequisites to use in my interactions with patients. In this role, I learned what it meant to be a part of a care team. I learned what it meant to work with a supervising physician. I learned how to work with an electronic medical records system. I learned how Physician Assistants (PA) interact with patients and providers.

I also learned that I don't want to be an MD or a DO. The most important part of getting into medicine for me is helping people. MDs and DOs get to do this of course but time and time again I hear patients saying "I just love my PA. They spend so much time with me. They know so much about my care but they also know about me as a person." This is what solidified my decision to pursue PA school. The skills that I have learned while working in primary care have been tremendous and will guide me as I enter the next level of my career in health care. However, the most important thing that I have learned while working in this setting, while taking courses in the evening, is that my passion for helping people, my passion for medicine, is truly inextinguishable. This is what my heart desires.

Commentary Essay 72

I'm starting with a few minor points. Your readers know what a CNA is, so just use the acronym. Your readers will also know what PA stands for. No need to explain. Don't capitalize physician assistant.

That being said, I like the opening lines of your essay. They're human and engaging. But after that, you lose focus. It's informative about everything except why you want to be a PA, and that's the most important thing to include. Getting to know patients and spending time with them is not unique to PAs. You really need to explain what about the profession specifically appeals to you, why it appeals to you, and what traits you have that make you a good candidate to be a PA. You can do this by talking about the work you've seen PAs do or work you've done with them. Generalities aren't helpful and make it seem as if you don't have an understanding of the profession.

You can cut a lot out of the first three paragraphs. That will leave you a lot of room to add the important information your essay lacks. Here's what I suggest for the first one:

"Whatever your heart desires, mine desires for you." This note was printed on the inside of a Valentine's Day card I received from an elderly patient during my second year as a CNA. I had cared for this patient nearly every day while working on my degree in International Studies. I had told him that my plan had been to go into medicine, but I had decided that I would rather help the underserved populace on a larger scale. One evening, I told him that I wasn't sure International Studies was right for me. He took my hand and said "Sarah, I need you to become a doctor so you can take care of me and people like me."

We writers are told to "kill your darlings." Nothing is sacred, not even your favorite words or stories. You'll have to do the same in your essay.

Also, take out the last line of your conclusion. It takes away from the strength of the sentence before it. You don't want to end your essay on a weak note.

Essay 73

This is my first draft and it needs a lot of work. It is over limit and I am not sure what to cut out. The last paragraph is also somewhat underwhelming. I would appreciate any input, thank you!

My decision to become a physician assistant cannot be traced to one defining moment. The need to become a PA developed over six years of health care experience. Experience that shaped my idea of healthcare and the role I wanted to play in the field. Growing from a vague inclination of wanting to "help people", my time as a CNA and a Medical Laboratory Scientist helped me to determine that I needed more than what those two career fields could offer individually. I need the patient interaction and emotional satisfaction of working as a CNA and the intellectual stimulation and challenge of correlating human disease with laboratory results. A career as a PA would allow me to unite the aspects I love about each field .

When I started my first job as a certified nursing assistant at a skilled nursing home I never expected that I would, or could do the job for the next five years. From my very first day forward, the work was emotionally draining, physically exhausting, and intellectually underwhelming. I saw the job as a necessary stepping stone, a rite of passage that would eventually lead to a better career. I thought, " I need the experience" having no concept at the time of what the word actually meant.

While countless interactions have contributed to my growth as a health care professional, one woman in particular stands out as the greatest influence. Her name was Kathryn. She was younger than most of the other residents at *** and she suffered from multiple sclerosis. Several of the other CNAs had cautioned me that she could be difficult to care for and that she was not shy about her distaste for some, or rather most, of the staff. Not to be dissuaded, I cared for her as best I could, though it was painfully obvious to the both of us how unfamiliar I was with her particular needs. Admittedly, she did not care for me in the beginning and it was disheartening for the both of us how unhappy she was. That being said I found myself more determined to be better for her. With time I became more efficient and was able to get her perfectly comfortable before I would leave her room. It seemed though to only make the slightest difference in her mood. She did however begin to open up to me about herself and the difficult life she had lead. As I would listen to her grievances, I had to stifle the urge to tell her , "its going to be ok" or "it will get better". I knew her well enough at this point to know that she did not find comfort in empty reassurances. When I did not know what to say, which was most of the time, I would sit and listen. When a reply was necessary, I would let her know that she meant a great deal to me and that I would do what I could for her. Over the years, her disposition improved considerably as we became more comfortable with each other. We both would laugh frequently and could speak frankly with each other, which she certainly appreciated.

Katheryn did not just need another care giver, she had plenty, what she wanted was a friend. She needed someone to confide in that would not criticize her for wanting to express her negativity. In turn I was able to provide better physical care for her by learning what she needed from me emotionally. Through her I was able to apply this skill to my interactions with other residents, each of whom needed something different from me. Not every person wants or needs a friend in their caregiver however, some simply want a competent practitioner, but it is the responsibility of that practitioner to make an honest effort to mold themselves into whatever their patients need them to be. This can only be accomplished given time and active listening, which is why I am dedicated to becoming a physician assistant family practitioner.

Upon Katheryn's passing, after almost five years of working as a CNA, I decided that I needed to pursue new opportunities and challenges. Despite all I had learned as a CNA, and the challenges I had to overcome, I found myself feeling deeply unsatisfied.

Wanting to experience the other side of the healthcare spectrum, I found myself drawn to laboratory medicine. The field not only requires knowledge of several areas, but is constantly changing with improvements in technology, providing endless opportunity for continuing education and new challenges. As a generalist in a hospital laboratory it is my responsibility to provide the practitioner with quality results with which they base their eventual diagnosis. This requires constant correlation of results from one department to the next. Chemistry, hematology, urinalysis, coagulation, microbiology, immunohematology, each provide insight to the overall health of the patient. An anomaly in one area has a ripple effect and will often effect the results of another area. Though exciting and mentally stimulating, I find myself yearning for more. I am never satisfied just providing the laboratory results. I often find myself following patient's progress, sometimes for weeks, and checking my own personal diagnosis of each patient against the practitioners. I not only want to play a more direct role in diagnosing the patient, but in their care overall. I have found that I desperately miss the patient interaction. After a year of working as a laboratory scientist, experiencing the field's benefits and shortcomings, I have decided that I will never be satisfied with a career in which I have such an indirect relationship with the patient. After careful consideration, I have found that to be truly fulfilled in my career is to join what I enjoy most about being a lab tech with what I loved about being a CNA. As a physician assistant in a family practice I would be able to foster long, quality relationships with patients while having the intellectual satisfaction of diagnosing and treating their ailments. Under the responsible supervision of a physician, I am determined to practice in the field that unites the best of each of my previous experiences.

Commentary Essay 73

You essay is over the 5000 CASPA character and space count by a little over 900. Despite its length, it's missing a key component — why you want to be a PA specifically, as opposed to any other healthcare professional. You could have long, quality relationships with patients and intellectual stimulation as a doctor or NP. You've got to include the PA specific information in your essay. If you've shadowed or worked with PAs, use real life examples from those experiences to make your points. When you add that additional information, you'll be able to form a stronger conclusion.

I worry that you describe your CNA work as follows: "From my very first day forward, the work was emotionally draining, physically exhausting, and intellectually underwhelming." Not only is it very negative but it seems inconsistent with your message in the rest of the essay, which is that you gained a lot from your five years as a CNA and even "loved" it. People don't know you — they first learn about you from your essay. So, cutting the negativity is a good place to start editing. The rest of that paragraph could be substantially cut, too.

The last paragraph should not be your conclusion. After what is now the last paragraph, you'll add a paragraph with the detailed, specific information about why you want to be a PA. Then you'll write a brief final paragraph for the conclusion.

Here's how I'd edit the last paragraph:

"Wanting to experience the other side of the healthcare spectrum, I found myself drawn to laboratory medicine. As a generalist in a hospital laboratory it is my responsibility to provide the practitioners with quality results with which they base their eventual diagnosis. Though exciting and mentally stimulating, I find myself yearning to play a more direct role in patient care. I often find myself following a patient's progress and checking my diagnosis against the practitioner's. After careful consideration, I know a truly fulfilling career will be one that joins what I enjoy most about being a lab tech with what I loved about being a CNA."

Now you have your lead-in to why you want to be a PA.

Essay 74

Kneeling in the pit house located in the Grand Staircase Escalante National Monument, grasping my trowel in one hand and using the brush in my other, I meticulously swept aside the dirt covering a charred human mandible, radius, and several cranial bones. Being an archaeologist was the most exciting career I could imagine because I love people and learning about their cultures. Both during and after my schooling to become an archaeologist I worked for several different programs to treat troubled kids and most recently with the mentally ill at the Utah State Hospital. It was during these work experiences that I came to realize that digging up the earthly remains of past peoples and cultures is fascinating, but archaeology is missing one key component. The people I work with are long dead and very likely couldn't care less what was done with the material remains of their existence, while the people of my own society and time are very much alive and in need of a lot of help.

Most nights during my shift on the Boys Youth Dorm at the Utah State Hospital, Darius asks me for a hug before bed and asks if I'll sit and talk with him for a couple of minutes. Unfortunately Darius has experienced a lot of awful things in his short 15 years; all have been inflicted upon him by those who should love him and protect him the most, his parents. One night Darius was having a particularly rough day. The other kids tease him and he can be frustrating for the staff to work with as he can be defiant and self-harms. As I sat next to him he bemoaned his fate, he was taken from his parents and placed in foster care and currently was being shuffled from one program to another before finally being placed in the mental hospital. He feels like there must be something wrong with him and that he is a terrible person because nobody wants him and his family doesn't come to visit him. I explained to Darius that being put into a facility like the hospital doesn't mean you are a bad person or that you've done something wrong, but rather he just needed a little help in getting life figured out and that we were there to help him. With tears streaming down his face he said to me, "You're just saying that because you're paid to, nobody here really cares about what happens to me." As I hugged him from the side and squeezed his shoulder I said, "Darius, they don't pay me enough to be here simply for the money. I care very much what happens to you and want to see you get out of here and go on to live a wonderful life. So you need to stop harming yourself, follow staff directions, and work to succeed in your program so that you can get out of here as soon as possible." With a smile he said, "Really you mean it?" "Yes, Darius, I'm here for you and I promise that life does get better. So cheer up, and don't hesitate to come to me when you need something," I gently replied.

I've had the chance to play this role for many kids having worked with at risk adolescents at a wilderness program in Idaho and two residential programs in Utah, as well as for the past 8 years at the Utah State Hospital. Working with psychiatrists, psychologist, social workers, nurses, and other psychiatric technicians like myself has shown me that I excel in an environment where I'm given autonomy in how I work with the patients, but we all have different strengths and qualities that we wield as a team to achieve the greatest amount of success in helping a patient. This is why I desire to continue my education and become a physician assistant. As I hang up my whip and leather jacket, I am grateful for the valuable tools my bachelor's degree in archaeology has given me. I have a strong work ethic, excel at looking at obscure clues to build the bigger picture, am sensitive to people of different cultures and races, and value the importance of looking at the past to understand the future.

Each new day working in health care brings not only new opportunities to serve, but also new ways to have my life shaped and molded as I work with new people who touch my life as much as I touch theirs. I am given such joy when a kid finds a little relief from a hug because they are feeling down or asks if I'm going to be working a double shift again tomorrow so that we can do another cooking group. Countless hours working with troubled kids and those of all ages suffering from illnesses of the mind has taught me that 1,000 years from now the only material remains that may exist of me for some archaeologist to dig up are the foundation of my house or the shards of my ceramic ware. However, helping people allows me to leave a legacy that will never fade. Like a stone dropped into the water of a tranquil lake, being a physician assistant will give me priceless opportunities to send ripples of change cascading down the history of a person's life and into the next generations of their children.

Commentary Essay 74

I really love this essay, but unfortunately, it doesn't give me a clue why you're picking the PA profession. The limited reasons you give for wanting to be a PA could apply to any number of healthcare or other professions. You need specific details about the PA profession and specifically why it appeals to you. You're a wonderful writer, so once you're on task, writing a great essay won't be a problem. Because of the essay's length, you'll need to shorten or eliminate parts. You could definitely shorten the story about Darius to make room for the necessary information.

One small technical item — contractions are disfavored in academic essays, so I recommend you don't use them in these.

Essay 75

"Permanence, perseverance and persistence in spite of all obstacles, discouragements and impossibilities: It is this; that in all things distinguishes the strong soul from the weak." Thomas Carlyle

My leadership, ambition, and commitment demonstrate qualifications for your Physicians Assistant program. In my past and previous work history, I have demonstrated exceptional work ethics. Always willing to go the extra mile, learn any new aspects of the organization, and to help out when necessary. I have taken on responsibilities that exceeded my job requirements, while understanding the importance such experiences and knowledge would provide me for long term success. At one particular point in my life, I decided to leave the comfort of a stable job to try my hand in the real estate market. Initially things went well until the market took a turn for the worse. Two years later I found myself out of a job. Denied unemployment and desperate for an avenue to support my four-year-old daughter, meanwhile searching hopelessly for a job. I subsequently created my own business, selling used goods at my local swap meet. When my personal merchandise was depleted, I extended my resources to the public and my social network of family and friends. This ambition and creativity sustained us financially until I was able to find steady employment. Throughout my adult life, I have consistently encountered adversities to the point of despair. However, my tenacious nature has allowed me to fulfill three most important accomplishments to date. My first accomplishment was completing a BSM (Bachelor of Science in Management) degree while continuing to work full time. Growing up in an underprivileged community, resources were limited and schools overpopulated. The occasion was rare when the notion of college was mentioned or made seemingly attainable. Being an average student, I went unrecognized, naïve to the limited resources and lacking the encouragement to prevail. Regardless of my environment I made the decision to change my fate and pursue something that was made obsolete my whole childhood. I was born into a family of five and I am the first to attend college. A second highlight in my life is one involving employment endeavors. I had less than three years of work experience when I was offered a job at The Spine Institute. I started as a file clerk, but through my excellent performance record and ambitious attitude, I successfully advanced to positions of increased responsibilities within a two-year period. At the age of twenty-one, I was offered an administrative position to assist a prestigious spine surgeon which I held for six years. It was then; that I was first introduced to PAs; and made the decision to pursue higher education and a new business venture. Finally, an accomplishment that was five years in the making and still in progress, is juggling the demands of fulltime employment, school, and single motherhood. I do owe a great deal of my success and ability to my strong circle of extended family and friends who have lent a hand when needed most, however with all the mental stresses; I always have every ounce of my being dedicated to a more further, higher and stronger pursuit. It is my hope that my achievements will pave the way for future generations including my daughter.

My career goal in becoming a physician's assistant was sparked when I was given the opportunity to help interrupt for our Spanish speaking patients. As I mentioned working in the Spine Center for six years, I noticed a pattern of our Latin patient's coming in with similar complaints, only after having visited a "Sobador" (These are unlicensed folk manual therapists; coming from the same socioeconomic background as many of their clients. These clients made up primarily of low-income families due to convenience of cost). I found myself constantly educating these patients via the doctor's advice on how such unsafe methods might have antagonized their existing diagnosis. Once a clear understanding was reached, patients were very grateful of said education and felt the need to share their own experience with family and friends. I felt personal satisfaction; having been a part of this educational bridge to the community. Realizing at that point, how vital a "team effort" can provide optimal patient care.

Obtaining a Physician's Assistant license would serve as an important educational tool when planning the establishment of low-cost clinics I hope to make available throughout underserved communities. My motivation to attend this program is to obtain a degree that will begin my path for a successful career.

At this point in my life, higher education will establish the confidence and spark my desire to achieve empowerment as a woman, mother, and service leader. This goes beyond a degree for me. Given this opportunity, I aspire to be the voice and reinforcement to those individuals with the culturally reinforced mentality that have allowed a subliminal wall of minority oppression to hold them back. Those like myself, at one point in life, who have been convinced that your socioeconomic status is inherited. Inherited based on the idea that once conceived into poverty, adversities come in abundance and will consume you; inevitably subjecting yourself to the "95" solution to survive.

After being in the medical field for over 15 years, I am well aware of the diverse nature in preventive medicine, and have obtained the necessary skills and compassion to adapt and meet the needs required of a PA to successfully assist the growing demand for a "Team". In the past two years I have dedicated my time to volunteer assignments ranging from community health outreach, a COACH for kids program raising health awareness to inner-city youth, and hospital ER assistance as applicable. I may not be a valedictorian, have an ideal GPA, or hold high test scores; instead I bring commitment and an undying motivational drive in which inspires me to sacrifice modest desires; to bring all my efforts into a rigorous science program.

Commentary Essay 75

You've had an amazing journey. But your essay doesn't do it justice because it doesn't maintain its focus. Nor does it demonstrate that you have a good understanding of the PA profession. For one, you call the profession by the wrong name in two different ways: Physician's Assistant and Physicians Assistant. It is physician assistant, not capitalized. These mistakes could easily cost you an interview. Nor do you explain why this profession is the one for you.

The main reason you give for wanting to be a PA is that it will help you when planning the establishment of low-cost clinics. I imagine a degree in Public Health or business would be much more helpful in that endeavor. Then you write, "My motivation to attend this program is to obtain a degree that will begin my path for a successful career." What career are you talking about if not that of a PA? At this stage, when you're applying to PA school, you're trying to convince the Admissions Directors and faculty that this is the profession for you.

You'll need to rewrite your essay. Read the ones posted here and the comments we've made to get an idea of where your focus needs to be.

Have people you work with in the medical profession, hopefully PAs read your essay after you revise it to see if you're on the right track.

Essay 76

The night of January 12, 2010 was the start of a defining chapter in my life. After delivering our patient to the emergency room I was completing my chart while my partner drove our ambulance back to base. I don't remember the song on the radio, but I remember the hysteria that broke through, reporting the 7.0 earthquake that just shattered Léogâne Haiti.

I had been to Haiti on medical missions twice in the preceding year with a physician team headed by a local pediatrician. He and his wife started a nonprofit organization that was in the middle of building a medical clinic in the remote location of Cayes, Haiti only miles from the epicenter of the earthquake. During the construction we held mobile clinics, which provided the only health care in that region of Haiti. These were often inside of schools, churches, or local orphanages.

My limited knowledge of building construction led me to believe that the destruction would be massive and the assistance needed would be immense. My first thoughts were of the many friends I had made during my short time in Haiti and I wondered if they were even still alive.

I knew that I would be receiving a phone call asking if I was able to deploy with the group yet again. I also knew that my answer would be a very complicated yes. My wife had just given birth to our first child just four months earlier. I grappled with the knowledge of enormous pain and suffering and I knew beyond a doubt that I was meant to help elevate and my responsibilities as a new father. Was I a horrible father because I could already leave my son to go help others? I don't know what frightened me more; the feelings of helplessness while people were suffering in Haiti or the feeling of letting my family down by leaving them.

In the end, my desire to teach my children to live their lives in the service of others won out and within six days I was in Haiti. I was beside myself. As a Marine infantryman who had served in Iraq, I knew what a war zone was. Seeing the devastation in Haiti was different. It looked like a war zone, but without the smell of ordinance or the sounds of weaponry. The destruction was no less real. We immediately started treating who we could with what we could. I delivered my first stillbirth under the light of a headlamp. I held a teenager's leg as an orthopedic surgeon amputated what remained after rubble crushed it.

A nurse and I had separated from the team to necessitate mobility in an effort to reach those who were completely unable to travel. We found a tent that was once staffed by Doctors Without Borders, whose waiting area was filled with patients to be seen. The first thing my eyes found was a four-year-old boy who had second and third degree burns to about sixty percent of his body. He just sat there whimpering. My feelings were a mixture of outrage and pity. Why was this child sitting there and suffering and no one was helping him? I then realized that there was in fact, no one else. There was only us. At this moment I was struck with the realization that I needed to further my education. If I wanted to do more, I would have to become more.

All of my life I've been infatuated with medicine. I knew early on that I lacked the patience and discipline necessary to be successful in college immediately after high school. I still needed a challenge, so I chose to enlist in Marine Corps Infantry. I knew that with the structure and disciple provided, I would learn the tools necessary to excel in whatever future endeavors I took on. After honorably serving in the Marine Corps I trained to become a paramedic and later, a firefighter. I enjoyed this line of work immensely, but felt something was missing. I was still on the front lines providing emergency medicine to those in need, but had a yearning to do more.

While working on the ground as a paramedic I had ample opportunities to interact with flight clinicians. These were the professionals that I looked up to and could utilize when patients were in need of immediate critical intervention and rapid transport to definitive care. It was their scope of practice and autonomy that first drew me to this field. After numerous discussions with these clinicians and hours of research I decided pursue this next step in my career path. This decision did not come without sacrifice. A move to Arizona as well as a new employer necessitated a significant reduction in benefits and pay. I didn't care about the money or the benefits. I wanted the ability to practice medicine. That's where my heart is. The autonomy was a bit overwhelming at first, but I instantly knew this was the right decision. I exceled quickly and within two years became a clinical educator.

I love being a flight paramedic and feel it is an honor to be among such an elite group of professionals. Certified flight paramedics make up approximately one percent of the paramedic population. This is not, however the extent of my career growth. My thirst for knowledge and responsibility has only grown stronger with my increased scope of practice and autonomy. The last two years have been a testament to my tenacity and commitment to becoming a physician assistant. While undergoing a divorce, I have nearly completed my bachelor's degree while maintaining a fulltime position as a flight paramedic and a Clinical Educator. During this time I created a ride along program for Arizona and New Mexico. This program works to create a stronger bond between the medical flight crew and hospital staff by allowing any medical clinician the chance to fly with the flight crew for a day. During this time they learn the capabilities of what flight medicine provides along with the challenges of delivering critical care medicine in the dynamic environment in which we work.

The achievements of the last few years however, have not been limited to only my career. As a single father my children have become a central part of my life. I have enjoyed volunteering at their school as well as actively participating in their numerous activities. Recently I have introduced them to my passion and respect for the outdoors. I have taken them rock climbing, exposed them to camping, taught them the basics of sailing, and have taken them on many excursions throughout the southwest.

While reinforcing my role as a father, I've also made time to return to Haiti multiple times on medical missions, volunteer for the Maricopa County Child Fatality Review Team which reviews pediatric fatalities on a monthly basis, competing in my first triathlon, breaking personal barriers as a rock climber, and organizing events for a local rock climbing group.

What draws me to a career as a physician assistant is multifaceted, but truly quite simple. I feel that physician assistants are afforded more time to interact with the patients and are not bridled with the politics and insurance requirements to the degree to which physicians are. Team collaboration is also appealing. My entire career has depended on collaborative efforts in some shape or fashion. I currently work with a flight nurse and the care we deliver to our patients is the result of a partnership, which is greater than the care either of us could provide single handedly. As a Clinical Educator I also collaborate with the physicians who make up our team of medical directors. Working side by side in cadaver labs, we teach flight clinicians the intricacies of invasive procedures including chest thoracotomies, surgical cricothyrotomies, oral intubations, escharotomies, intraosseous access, central line access, etc. Teaching the human patient simulator lab also gives me the opportunity to refine these procedures and skills. Another draw to the field is the diversity in which physician assistants are able to practice medicine. I have a great passion for cardiology, emergency and critical care medicine and know that I would be an asset to all of these specialties.

It is not my experiences that make me a great candidate for physician assistant school, but the experiences that have shaped who I am today. I am an individual capable of handling highly stressful situations, collaborating with multidisciplinary fields, and advocating for me patients all with goal of safely providing the best patient care possible.

Commentary Essay 76

You've been through some incredible experiences. But you can't write about all of them here. Your essay is 8,272 characters (spaces count, too), and the limit is 5,000.

Due to the length of the essay, it's difficult to give you any advice that would be helpful.

Take out anything that isn't absolutely essential, things like, "During this time they learn the capabilities of what flight medicine provides along with the challenges of delivering critical care medicine in the dynamic environment in which we work", and "Working side by side in cadaver labs, we teach flight clinicians the intricacies of invasive procedures including chest thoracotomies, surgical cricothyrotomies, oral intubations, escharotomies, intraosseous access, central line access, etc." Scrutinize every word, and you'll find plenty of places to cut.

Essay 77

Throughout my life, I have used my challenges and shortcomings to motivate me. I was diagnosed with kidney disease when I was 15. By the time I was 22 years old, I went to dialysis daily, had many symptoms from kidney failure, was working part-time, and was going to school full time. I had a lot on my plate but I saw the ultimate goal. I wanted a career in healthcare but even in my junior year of college, I was not sure which direction I wanted to take. It was finally a life changing experience that made me seriously think of pursuing a career as a physician assistant.

In March 2015, I received a call that a kidney was available for me. So many emotions rushed through me but I knew this was my ticket to a new healthy life. Throughout the process, physician assistants were there for me to talk to daily. They were caring and paid attention to my every need. PAs made up most of my postoperative transplant team and it really surprised me how much command they had in the decision-making process. I inquired about a career as a physician assistant before but I was also interested in other professions, which made me unsure of my decision.

My experience as a kidney transplant recipient has truly helped me in my decision to pursue this profession. As a patient, I appreciated that I had someone with medical training that I can talk to multiple times a day. I was able to communicate to my surgeon and nephrologist through my physician assistant when I had more specific concerns. When I had to return to the hospital for complications with the surgery, a physician assistant met me in one of the busiest emergency rooms in NYC just to assure me that a room in the transplant unit would soon be available. The feeling of reassurance that they provided for me during one of the most difficult periods of my life was appreciated and I want to be able to reciprocate that feeling to patients as a physician assistant.

One of the few calls I will always remember as an EMT is my first infant death. Everything around me was in slow motion as I was assessing the situation but when his small body was laid into my hands; my adrenaline went into over drive. As *Amari lay like a doll, I started to resuscitate him while my partner was in hysterics and the "newbie" was in shock. It was almost like tunnel vision; I couldn't concentrate on anything else but his breath. As I continued to resuscitate Amari, bruises slowly started to show on his soft skin. How can anyone do this to a child? Transporting *Amari to the hospital seemed like an eternity, while the paramedics pumped medications into his tiny veins. My tunnel vision stopped as soon as I heard the bloodcurdling cry of his mother as the ambulance arrived at the hospital.

Weeks later at his funeral, I was surprised to discover Amari's organs were donated and helped many people. To reassure his mother, I shared my story of needing a kidney. I explained to her that those that were blessed with his organs have waited so long for a new lease on life and that Amari definitely served his purpose here on Earth. "Those were the words I needed to hear", she said. I was happy to provide her comfort by sharing my experiences.

This area of healthcare has taught me how to work under conditions of high stress, allowing me to think independently in a versatile environment. It has also educated me on the importance of life and the benefits preventative care provides. Most of the emergency situations I come across are avoidable and have shown me the significance of promoting beneficial routines while discouraging the harmful. I was also able to relate to some of my patients health issues and sometimes was able to share personal experiences. Thus being a PA will not only give me the ability to positively influence peoples' lives, but also allow me to use my personal experiences to become more relatable to the patient.

I have been exposed to many areas of healthcare and medicine. I have experienced the patient side by having kidney disease and receiving a kidney transplant. As an EMT, I have experienced patient care and have had calls that have affected me for the rest of my life and have shaped me to be a better healthcare provider. I have participated in medical education programs such as SMDEP (Summer Medical and Dental Education Program) that have exposed me to various areas in medicine and demonstrated how healthcare providers can work as a team and individually. Volunteering in the emergency room at a trauma center showed me the fast paced environment that I am used to but mainly as an observer. Seeing how the step-by-step process of saving someone's' life is remarkable. And my most recent occupation as a 911 dispatcher has taught me a different side to providing patient care. Even though I cannot physically see my patient, I must be able to pick up cues and efficiently provide the best care through my words and resources.

As I embark on this new journey in becoming a physician assistant, I have realized with my experiences that I want to be remembered not by my title, but what I did with my title to help people in a positive manner. This message has persevered in many areas of my life and I foresee that continuing in a career as a physician assistant.

Commentary Essay 77

I can tell you've spent a lot of time on this. Overall it's well done. You've done a good job of showing your experience and qualifications in an interesting way.

Watch for long (bordering on run-on) sentences, which are prevalent throughout. Vary the sentence length — take out the "and" to make two or even three separate sentences. Be careful about your word choices. They can make or break an essay.

This is one example of a long sentence with word choices that could be better: As an EMT, I have experienced patient care and have had calls that have affected me for the rest of my life and have shaped me to be a better healthcare provider.

First, I don't think you meant to say "calls that have affected me for the rest of my life." I think you meant "calls that will affect me for the rest of my life." See how it looks when edited: "As an EMT, I have delivered patient care. I have had calls that will affect me for the rest of my life and have made me a better healthcare provider." The word "shaped" doesn't work the way you used it.

On the grammar side, punctuation comes before quotation marks. In your essay, this sentence should read, "Those were the words I needed to hear," she said.

One part I found awkward was the part about Amari being transported. It all has a negative feeling — the use of tunnel vision adds to it. I'd edit it as follows: As Amari lay like a doll, I started to resuscitate him. All my concentration focused on his breath. As I continued to resuscitate him, bruises slowly started to show on his soft skin. How can anyone do this to a child? Transporting him to the hospital seemed like an eternity, while the paramedics pumped medications into his tiny veins. My concentration broke when I heard the blood-curdling cry of his mother as the ambulance arrived at the hospital."

Essay 78

During my 2008 graduation commencement ceremony a classmate said, "You go to school here? I thought you only worked for Chartwells [our food service provider]. You were always there!" I was hurt that he did not recognize me as an academic peer.

Even though I did not have the social life of my classmates, the time I spent working outside of school was not in vain. As an undergraduate I had to care for myself as well as my youngest brother, Tyler.

My mother was not prepared for the birth of her fourth child, and because of that Tyler was born chronically ill. Compelled to ensure the baby's health, I decided to help raise him. This was not an easy endeavor as I had to interact with multiple doctors during countless visits, discuss and understand his diagnoses, and ask critical questions. Because he suffered from constant lung infections I spent a great deal of time researching medications and their side effects in an effort to assist his breathing. Then I would examine his symptoms with my mother and figure out if Tyler was making progress or having a setback. Throughout this entire process I also learned the importance of not letting my emotions and frustrations compromise my ability to improve his health. Medicine is not what I had originally thought it to be and through my experiences I came to understand that it is an intricate process that is not as black and white as it may seem. The dynamics and process in caring for Tyler inspired me to practice medicine.

My undergraduate years were not spent at parties or on wild spring break trips, they were spent travelling to NYC to see pulmonologists and visiting my sick brother. In my sophomore year my brother's health was at his worse; the amount of infections he caught was increasing and trips to the Emergency Room were becoming more frequent. My focus shifted completely from trying to earn my degree to caring for my brother. However, this would mean working multiple jobs to support him. I became a NYS EMT and volunteered at the on campus daycare site for 3 years. These experiences, which ranged from responding to car accidents to interacting with parents, were invaluable especially if medicine was something I would pursue in my future. My undergraduate grades are a reflection of my choice, not of my academic ability. I graduated from college and began my Master's degree in 2008. My brother's health deteriorated to the point where he could no longer live with my mother and I decided that he needed to live with me. I became a full time parent while simultaneously succeeding in graduate school and earning a higher GPA.

Since 2008, I have worked for the University at Albany as a professional staff member for the Department of Residential Life providing services for the students who live on campus. When a promotional opportunity was presented to me I started evaluating if I wanted to continue working in Higher Education. While I have enjoyed many aspects of my work, such as interacting with students during some of the most personal and difficult moments in their college careers, my passion was not fulfilled. Medicine was the piece that was missing. It was also around this time that Tyler had improved to the healthiest he had ever been in his whole life. I decided to focus on a career in medicine. I was excited about my decision, but felt a little uncertain. To quell my doubts I left my job in Higher education and began working in a local hospital, and immersed myself in the job.

As roles in medicine became clear through my 2013 medical mission work in Haiti and work at the hospital as a Patient Care Associate in a Surgical Neurosciences Intensive Care Unit. It was clear in my interactions with patients, their families, physicians, and the nurses, I found a sense of satisfaction. This is where I can fully use my experiences with Tyler to make an impact by not only providing medical care for patients with acute and chronic diseases but also through educational evaders such as training new staff. After these realizations I knew Physician Assistant was the professional road I wanted to take to practice medicine. Physician Assistant allows for my diverse background to be fully utilized to benefit a medical team in all aspects of patient care.

Looking back on my life, I do not regret the decisions I have made in caring for my brother. While difficult at times, this road has led to more life experiences than I ever thought possible. I truly believe that had I not raised a sick child I would not be an attentive practitioner. My experiences have given me the determination and maturity to purse medicine at a professional level. I can now say that I am able to take the Physician Assistant Professional Oath because I understand what it means to be passionate, to work hard, and be wholly dedicated to helping another person have the best outcome possible but also knowing that it takes many to achieve that goal.

Commentary Essay 78

The opening is not as strong as it should be. No one cares if your feelings are hurt (sorry to say). Here's a more positive way of approaching your essay:

"My undergraduate years were not spent at parties or on wild spring break trips, they were spent travelling to NYC visiting my sick brother, Tyler and seeing his pulmonologists. Even though I did not have the social life of my classmates, the time I spent working outside of school was not in vain."

You do a good job of explaining why your grades suffered. But you never address specifically why you wish to become a PA as opposed to any other medical professional. That's a must according to every Admissions Director and faculty member I've spoken with. You make a few general statements that could actually apply to many other professions. Have you shadowed PAs? Worked with them? Give some specific detail about what appeals and why.

There are places to cut so you can add this information. You've seen how that can work in the revised first paragraph. It uses all your words in a concise way.

Here's another example. Your original paragraph, "I was excited about my decision, but felt a little uncertain. To quell my doubts I left my job in Higher education and began working in a local hospital, and immersed myself in the job," would read "I left my job in higher education and immersed myself in a job at a local hospital." All the other details are unnecessary, and can bog down the message you're trying to deliver.

By the way, higher education is not capitalized.

Essay 79

The most exciting experiences of growing up as biology teacher's daughter were getting to play with the skeletons in lab, taking home the lab rats for the summer, playing with cells and micro organelles made of clay, throwing project planets at my brother, among many more things. Inquisitive, curious, and satiated for answers, it was becoming of me as a scientist. In fifth grade, there was a discolored mass on my left breast that needed to be removed. The surgeon used local anesthetics for numbing while my eyes were glued to my mom for comfort. However, once numb, my curious nature to watch her do the invasive removal took over. It was the so interesting to see the mass in the doctors forceps and to know that a biopsy was going to be conducted to answer my question: what was that lump in me?! To our relief it was a benign tumor, to me it just looked like chicken fat. Nonetheless, my career coupled with my fascination in a medical profession was being impressed upon. There are many other experiences that have directed, shaped, and concluded my heart upon being a PA.

Ambitiousness, determination, self-disciplined, accomplished the title of salutatorian of my graduating high school class. Attending MSU for college was the biggest growth spurt this 4'11 girl had. Being predisposed to alcoholism changed my priorities my first few semesters of college. My MSU transcript reflects this especially in comparison to my ECTC and UK transcripts. However, the most worthwhile things are acquired through struggle and perseverance. Becoming a member of Alcoholics Anonymous gave me a strength unbeknown to me at twenty years old. Compassion was taught to me and I never thought I could possess the amount that I now have. Jewel sings a song that says "dark is dark so the stars have a place to shine" which is an understatement to the feeling I have for life, for light, for inspiration. I sat across a table from a recovered alcoholic who shared her experience, strength, and hope with me with intentions I would do the same for another sufferer. And so it begun, working with sick people, becoming selfless, is where I found myself.

I know I could never requite the life AA has granted me but there are certain things within my power I can do to give back to my community. KCYPAA (Kentucky Conference of Young People in AA) was held in Lexington 2012 and the position I held was Arts and Graphics Chair. Our mission was to "raise the bottoms" of young people and to show others how to have fun sober; it was an amazing experience to watch people come together for a common purpose. I have also served as a GSR (Group Service

Representative) which means I represent my homegrown for the business of AA. I have given my testimony countless times, served as a grapevine representative, given ladies rides to meetings, chaired meetings, and simply door greeted. However, sitting with another woman, giving her time and service to help her is something that has left a lasting impression, and again emphatically reassures me on becoming a PA.

Other than working with alcoholic women I have been privileged to care for people with Alzheimer's. It has had its humorous moments, tragic moments, and challenging moments. However, my care transcends to their family and loved ones because they suffer equally. Therefore, my drive to provide outstanding care was enhanced beyond what they eye could see. My mind goes to the love and care I would want for my parents. I have also had the amazing opportunity to go on a medical missionary trip to Mexico with PA students and PAs. We set up a clinic in a drug rehabilitation center where I was able to connect with some newly sober people while taking their blood pressure. Although I wasn't a medical provider, I provided what I could which was hope and dignity.

Shadowing a variety of PAs has allowed me to reaffirm my commitment of becoming a PA. Getting a medical history, performing a physical, diagnosing, and treating the patient is a method that complements my mind as a scientist. I enjoyed watching the collaborative work between the PAs and physicians to provide the patient the ultimate care. Becoming a PA allows flexibility in choosing a career path. For example, I am highly interested in neurosurgery but my experience in geriatrics has captured my heart. The freedom of being able to be in different fields throughout my life excites me. The idea of having to specialize in one field and do 37 years of residency, plus the excess debt, is something that I am not interested in. Being in the prePA club and a member of KAPA has taught me that laws are changing to better PAs and I want to be apart of that growth. My hope is become the best possible me, to be believed in, so that, in turn, I can believe in others.

Commentary Essay 79

Congratulations on your sobriety, and for your commitment to giving to the community. You clearly have great empathy, a quality that helps make a great PA.

Your essay makes some good points, but gets off topic, starting from the beginning. Admissions Directors and faculty have said they don't want to know about early childhood experiences. Your opening, which is where you really want to grab your reader's attention, starts with information they're not interested in. I recommend taking out almost the whole first paragraph. It's too remote to be of real use. It would be different if you continued to have health issues, but it doesn't sound like it.

You could start your essay by saying something about having a curious nature, which played out when you had a tumor removed in the fifth grade, and to everyone's surprise, you were more interested in watching the surgery than afraid of the pain. Then you could write how your scientific curiosity has remained, but it was your life experiences that brought you to the place in life where you're applying to PA school.

Some of your writing is awkward. For example, these two sentences:

"Ambitiousness, determination, self-discipliness accomplished the title of salutatorian of my graduating high school class," and "Therefore, my drive to provide outstanding care was enhanced beyond what they eye could see." (I'm ignoring the typo "they" instead of "the" but you can't ignore them when you submit your final essay). I'm not sure what you mean by this either: "I know I could never requite the life AA has granted me." I think you're trying way too hard to make the essay sound formal. The writing is much more clear when you're just being yourself and writing like you normally talk.

You focus far too much on your AA experiences. The details are not as important to the essay as you might think. You can combine the second two paragraphs into one. The points to make are that your drinking impacted your grades, that not only are you in recovery, but you've done significant work to help others. That explains any academic issues you had and shows your compassion.

The main focus of your essay should be your work with Alzheimer's patients and your shadowing experiences. Can you give examples by describing actual work with patients to show how you've helped patients and their families rather than just making general statements like these: "However, my care transcends to their family and loved ones because they suffer equally. Therefore, my drive to provide outstanding care was enhanced beyond what the eye could see. My mind goes to the love and care I would want for my parents."

I'm certain in caring for Alzheimer's patients, you've had emergency situations, stressful incidents, had to work with other care professionals. Describe a situation with a patient that shows what you mean by "It has had its humorous moments, tragic moments, and challenging moments." How did you respond? Did you learn you have the ability to deal with emergencies? Or work with other medical professionals? Did you learn that it often takes time to figure out what a patient needs? These are things you should be talking about.

Do the same with what you've witnessed when you were shadowing a PA.

You have many strengths, that much is clear. In this essay, you want to emphasize them in the context of why you want to be a PA, and how your personal (not necessarily clinical) skills will make you a good PA.

I would always emphasize the positive. So leave out that you don't want to spend seven years studying to be a doctor.

Don't use exclamation points, and never use "?!."

I know this may sound like a lot to tackle, but you've already over-come a challenge that many people never come close to doing. I am confident you can tackle this one, too.

Essay 80

Selfless giving and the feeling that comes with it is the best feeling in the world. It takes a certain kind of person to possess these qualities and to never expect anything in return, beyond knowing they have given of themselves unconditionally. There are many levels of this character trait and those fortunate enough to have it know how rewarding it is. It knows no difference between age, skin color, religion, or the likelihood of reciprocation. It is with great certainty that I feel Physician Assistants embody this quality.

"Ugh, yes, that was the nastiest junk I've ever had to drink!" exclaimed my study participant. "I hear it's not the most pleasant stuff," I said, mimicking the face he had made. I had just recruited Mr. Walker for a research study and he and his wife were looking a bit nervous. I had been working in a GI clinic as a clinical research assistant for over a year and had met people from all walks of life who were coming in for their first colonoscopy. Most of my study participants were over 50 years old and having their procedure as a preventive screening. Mr. Walker was quite different. Mr. Walker was a 36 year old man whose younger brother had passed away a few months earlier from colon cancer. His wife was on the verge of tears as I explained the study to them. She was so afraid for her husband and he was trying his best to be strong for the both of them. I assured them that he would be getting excellent care and that they were doing the right thing having this procedure, no matter the outcome. I explained how the procedure would go and how the doctor would remove anything worrisome. As the nurse took him back and his wife returned to the waiting room, I did not know if my explanation eased their minds, but at least they had a better idea of what was going to happen. I had only talked with them for a few minutes, but my heart hurt for them and the unknown outcome they were facing. I wanted so badly for Mr. Walker to be okay; I held my breath as I watched his procedure. Fortunately, he did not have a single polyp, much less any evidence of cancer. When I saw the Walkers as they were leaving the clinic, the look of relief was written all over their faces. A weight had been lifted from them. Although I had only met them that day, I felt like a weight had been lifted from me as well. Even though I was able to give them information and console them, I longed to do more. This is just one instance of the many interactions I have been fortunate to have with patients and that feeling cannot be replaced.

I did not always want to be a Physician Assistant; in fact, I had not even heard of the profession until several years ago. I have always wanted to be helpful and appreciated, but my initial focus was on helping animals. Eventually the desire to work in the healthcare field found me and it has motivated and inspired me more than any other career I have considered. The feeling I get when I help someone in any way is like no other, and it makes me crave it more and more. I am fascinated by science, biology and the human body. Of my experiences working with various healthcare professionals, including doctors, nurses, nurse practitioners, and physician assistants, I find that physician assistants have a more personal relationship with their patients. This seems to hold true whether the interaction is brief, like in the emergency department, or lasting, such as in a primary care setting. I am meant to help others – it has been programmed into me. I was raised to put others before myself and I take great joy in knowing I have helped someone in some way, no matter how big or small.

Commentary Essay 80

I love the opening to the second paragraph. In fact, the whole second paragraph is really good except where you say you mimicked Mr. Walker. It sounds as if you're making fun of him or being snotty, and I know neither is true.

The second paragraph should be your first paragraph, and the opening paragraph you have now should be deleted. It's filled with generalizations and platitudes, what I call "throat clearing." You're just getting ready to write what you need to write. It doesn't say a word about you, which is the whole point of a personal essay.

Normally I'm telling people their essays are too long. Yours is too short. It doesn't have any specifics about your work with PAs (I assume you've shadowed or interacted with them in your work because you mention them) and why you specifically want to become a PA. Having a personal relationship with a patient is not specific to PAs. Doctors, nurses, CNAs all do, too. It's not enough to say that's why you want to become one.

Are there specific cases you can describe that exemplifies what you appreciate about the PA profession? If so, write about those. I know you have the skills to do it by the wonderful story you told about the Walkers.

Here's what you want your readers to know — that you understand what the PA profession entails and that you have personal traits that are compatible with the profession. You haven't said a lot about either.

In your third paragraph, you should leave out that you wanted to work with animals. That isn't key to your essay. These sentences also are general: "Eventually the desire to work in the healthcare field found me and it has motivated and inspired me more than any other career I have considered. The feeling I get when I help some-one in any way is like no other, and it makes me crave it more and more." Instead of writing these generalities, write what actually motivated you. There was a turning point where it clicked. Was there a patient in particular? Or was it the culmination of a number of experiences? If so, mention those.

By the way, it's very passive to say "the desire to work in the healthcare field found you." It sounds like you ended up interested in healthcare by chance. I don't think you need a sentence like that, anyway, but if you do, make it active — My desire to work in healthcare motivated me . . . etc.

Essay 81

Throughout life we will be impacted by people. Friends, family, and strangers will subtly influence the direction of our lives. The first time I noticed the impact people can make, was in an unfamiliar part of town, in a foreign country. I stepped off the subway in Shanghai, China and with every step towards my destination, anticipation rose. I finally reached the building I was looking for, a small homeless shelter. A Chinese man opened the door. As expected, but with little disappointment, he told me he did not speak English. As he led me into a room, hazy with cigarette smoke, he introduced himself as Tian. I scanned the room, sat down with him at a table filled with men and started to learn about their lives. After graduating college, I spent two years living in China working with a Christian mission's organization. My job was to talk with college students about what was important to them; what their beliefs were and what shaped their worldviews. During that time, I learned a lot about people and what drove them. I cherish most the opportunity to learn how to interact with a variety of people. Especially, people whose culture and background is incredibly different from my own. The people I have met and their stories drive me towards a career as a physician assistant (PA).

While I was in China I had a friend who volunteered at a homeless shelter. She invited me to help lead an art therapy class for the shelter's residents. The long term goal was to help teach people to express themselves and gain marketable skills through art. Due to my inability to speak Chinese fluently, my lack of technical art skills, and my inexperience working with the homeless, it proved to be my mountain to climb. I continued going to the shelter and helping to the best of my abilities. The more time I spent with them, the more I realized that even the smallest efforts can help people in great ways. This is something that I believe holds true in the PA to patient relationship.

Many of the men at the shelter were there because they were sick. They had no one to help or care for them. We all understand that poor health affects our quality of life. Working as a nursing assistant, I see just how true this statement can be. On my first day of clinical training, a woman named Gina asked me to get her ready to go home. After checking with the staff and realizing she was on hospice care, I had to break the news to her that she would not be able to go home that day. She started to cry, but there was nothing I could do. I held her hand and let her know that I cared. As a PA I would continue to bring dignity and kindness to my patients.

Having shadowed a PA in I saw the effect one person, who cares, can have on an individual. Relationships are built between the PA and their patient, over the smallest period of time. The PA, I had the privilege to watch, spent his time educating and explaining, to patients, their different diagnoses and helping then come to terms. If the PA was unsure he went to his team and asked for a consultation. He believed that, "The health of one is the health of us all". Watching him work with this attitude and seeing the great patients responses, affirmed my passion to become a PA who takes charge and provides the best care.

The choice to pursue a career in medicine is clear, for me. I want to live not for myself, but doing something for the greater good. My story will be about the part I play in the lives of others, and what I can accomplish to help them thrive. My desire is to work both in primary care and to take part in medical missions where people might not otherwise receive care. No matter what, my life's story will not be just my own. The lives we lead will have an impact on those we meet. My legacy will be providing care, both emotional and health to my patients as a PA.

Commentary Essay 81

There are some excellent parts of your essay. The ending is quite good, and sums up everything you've written well.

You spend too much time on your China experience, though. You could easily consolidate it into one paragraph to summarize the points you make — that you've learned to interact with people of different cultures, that you perform well and can adapt to difficult conditions, that giving and that kindness are critical to good health care. For example, look at the first and second sentences of your opening paragraph. The second in particular, "The first time I noticed the impact people can make, was in an unfamiliar part of town, in a foreign country," makes a promise to the reader. Yet, you never specifically talk about anyone who impacted you or how you impacted others in that whole first paragraph. The Admissions faculty won't particularly care what your job was there, or that you learned a lot about people. Most of it is very general and could go. The same is true of the second paragraph.

The area where you need to write more is your work experience as a nursing assistant and shadowing PAs. Use those experiences as your examples to show that not only do you understand the role of the PA, but that it is the right profession for you and you are right for the profession. Be specific, using examples.

Essay 82

Life is not about how much you receive, but about how much you give back. Helping others gives our life purpose and makes the world around us a better place. My Physician Assistant (PA) said, "The most important lesson about becoming a PA is that patients always comes first and the license comes second." This philosophy will embody the type of PA I want to become. My desire as a PA is to give high quality health care to the underprivileged population.

When I arrived at Texas Tech, I thought I wanted to become a Physical Therapist. My reasoning for wanting to become a Physical Therapist is for my love of sports and exercise. Even though I loved learning about Physical Therapy, I wanted to do more. My desire to become a PA came from studying abroad in Spain. After two months in Spain, I became very ill and contracted the flu. I needed to see a doctor and receive medication. I was very nervous entering the doctor's office because I had heard bad stories about socialized medicine. However, when I entered the doctor's office he alleviated all of my fears. He was very polite, and we had the opportunity to speak broken Spanish and English to each other. Despite our language barrier, I could sense his compassion. The doctor's kindness inspired me to become a PA and to treat every patient with the same compassion that the doctor showed me.

When I came back to America, I wanted to prescribe medicine and see a variety of patients, something PT can't offer. I started doing research and discovered the PA profession in the counselor office. After I graduated from Texas Tech University, I shadowed PA Nancy Lounds. Nancy runs a free clinic for uninsured students in the Clear Lake ISD and Dickinson area. At this clinic I observed Nancy making diagnoses and prescribing medicine. During my shadowing hours I was able to check patient's vitals, talk to UTMB PA students, answer phone calls, speak Spanish with patients, and helped Nancy with paperwork. Watching Nancy work with the uninsured population was an eye opening experience. I learned that high quality health care in this country is a huge problem for the uninsured population. The rising cost of health care every year makes it almost impossible for the underprivileged to afford any type of health care.

The route I would like to go as a PA would be helping the uninsured population in primary care. Being a primary care PA would be the perfect occupation for me because I like to be challenged intellectually and I love to teach. Being a PA is not all about making diagnoses and prescribing treatments; it is also educating patients about their problem. In order to have a good patient to PA relationship, teaching needs to be involved. I want to create an atmosphere where the patient can ask me questions without being intimidated. My love for teaching stems from tutoring high school kids at Bay Area Learning Center. I enjoy teaching because I never stop learning and I enjoy being challenged intellectually. I believe that the PA profession will give me the opportunity to continue teaching and learning for a lifetime.

The medical field is constantly growing, and I would like to grow along with this field so that I can learn on a daily basis. I want to be a PA because I want patients to learn from me, and I also want to learn from my patients in a collaborative effort. Being a PA will be a rewarding occupation for me because I have the opportunity to experience something different on a daily basis. The PA profession fits my personality because my personality is always growing and never static. The lessons that I have learned from Nancy, study abroad, tutoring and Texas Tech make me well equipped to be successful in the PA program. I believe that my hard work, a desire to learn, and self-confidence are the tools that will make me the best Physician Assistant that I can be.

Commentary Essay 82

Your essay has a lot of heart, but it's presented in a way that reads more like a report rather than an essay that flows. While you did a good job of transitioning from one sentence to the next for the most part (something a lot of people struggle with), the way you do it is a bit stilted. The second paragraph is a good example of the concern I have with your style. If you were to rewrite it in a more story-like way, this is what I'd suggest:

"When I arrived at Texas Tech, I thought I wanted to become a physical therapist — it combined my love of sports and exercise with my love of healing and helping people. Even though I loved learning about physical therapy, a personal experience while studying abroad in Spain showed me it would not be enough. Two months into the semester, I contracted the flu and became very ill.

I knew I needed to see a doctor, but I was very nervous about it because I had heard negative stories about socialized medicine. However, the doctor alleviated all of my fears. We had the opportunity to speak broken Spanish and English to each other, and despite our language barrier, I could sense his compassion. He prescribed the proper medication and within two days I felt great. When I came back to America, I wanted to do the same for others, something PT could not offer."

Also in your opening paragraph, rather than making a general philosophical statement, make it personal to you: "I believe that life is not . . ." A couple of other things. Most professions are not capitalized (including physician assistant and physical therapy) unless used in a formal name. Also, contractions are disfavored in academic essays, so don't use them in these personal statements. Finally, anyone reading these essays knows that PA stands for physician assistant, so no need to put the acronym in parentheses.

Essay 83

"We have an MI being brought in by EMS, be prepared to document everything that goes on in that room, from the medications given to the time the patient is under critical care." The doctor told me as we rushed to get ourselves situated to care for the incoming patient. As the patient was wheeled into the room the physician and the physician assistant immediately took over to try to bring the patient back to stable condition. "Give one shot of epinephrine!" The doctor yelled trying to get a heartbeat. Twenty minutes had passed and the patient was still unresponsive. I stood in the corner anxiously staring at the cardiac monitor, wishing I could do more to help. The physician was unable to intubate the patient, it had been too late. As the doctor called time of death, my heart plummeted into my stomach; I was not prepared for this.

I did not always know I wanted a career in medicine, however my desire to "do more" pushed me towards healthcare. I began college believing that becoming a doctor was my only option. To further acquaint myself with the medical profession, I started shadowing Dr. Passi, a physician specializing in cardiology. Shadowing Dr. Passi deepened my interest in medicine; I realized my desire to want to interact with patients on a daily basis. I initially became familiar with the physician assistant profession my sophomore year of college, however, I learned the true role of a PA when I began to shadow Lara West, a PA specializing in Emergency Medicine. Lara became my role model and my shadowing experience influenced my decision to become a PA. Shadowing Lara sparked my critical thinking and taught me how to evaluate a patient holistically. I learned the various responsibilities of a PA such as diagnosing, treating, educating and prescribing medications under the supervision of a physician. I also learned about the flexibility PAs have when switching between different specialties. Being able to compare the roles of a physician and a PA in a medical setting broadened my interest in the PA career. I learned the vital role PAs play in the healthcare team to provide quality patient care by working together with their supervising physician. It was during my shadowing experience I saw myself as a future physician assistant.

I have prepared myself for the challenges of PA school and the PA career through my academic and professional experiences. Although I struggled balancing my classes and extracurricular activities during my freshmen and sophomore year, my academic improvement from junior to senior year highlights my ability to reevaluate my work habits. I learned to use my time efficiently by prioritizing activities and studying actively which will help me succeed through a PA program.

Receiving rejections from PA schools was initially very disappointing, but upon reevaluating my application, I realized I had much to learn. I continued working as a medical assistant where I gained more experience interacting with patients. I also began working as an Emergency Department scribe which exposed me to the daily responsibilities of a physician and PA. As a scribe, I became the PA's helping hand by efficiently completing patient charts as they examined patients. Listening to numerous patient interviews has trained me to focus on pertinent information of the patient's complaint and has also made me proficient at comprehending medical terminology. By working with doctors and PAs on a daily basis, I have witnessed the transition of healthcare to a more team based approach. Working as a scribe has instilled in me a sense of responsibility, as my charts are the sole evidence of a patient's visit. Among the fast pace environment of the ED, I not only learned to work efficiently, but I gained the skills necessary to interact with patients and medical staff in various circumstances which is something I will be doing as a PA. To broaden my knowledge of the PA career, I began shadowing PAs in urgent care and internal medicine. I witnessed the difference in practice of PAs in various medical settings. Throughout these experiences, I have become familiar with taking medical histories, performing patient physical examinations, performing medical procedures, medical decision making and patient disposition. My clinical experiences have given me the interpersonal skills necessary to become a successful PA student and PA.

From shadowing to listening to a patient's chief complaint, I have gained a true understanding of the role and responsibilities of a PA. My various clinical and volunteer experiences have deepened my interest in medicine and desire to become a PA. As a reapplicant, I have seen growth in myself. My experiences have shaped me into a responsible and mature person, and have prepared me for the training required to become a PA. With confidence, I can now say that I am ready for the challenges that will come my way as a PA student and a future PA, and I am very excited to begin this new chapter of my life.

Commentary Essay 83

First, you did an excellent job of covering your progress since being rejected the first go-around. That will impress your readers.

Your opening paragraph is attention grabbing and that's good. (There's a grammar error, by the way. When you end the quoted dialog in the first sentence, you'll have a comma after "care" instead of a period). But the paragraph doesn't lead anywhere. It ends on a serious note that requires an insight somewhere in the essay or it's pointless. We are never given that insight.

You need to break up your second paragraph. Readers need a white space to give their eyes a rest.

If you're looking to cut, you have lots of opportunities. Here's how I would edit the first two sentences of the second paragraph:

I began college believing that becoming a doctor was my only option. I started shadowing a physician specializing in cardiology. Shadowing Dr. Passi deepened my interest in medicine; I realized my desire to interact with patients on a daily basis.

That cuts a lot of words and delivers the same message. I suggest you go through and take out what's not critical. That way you'll keep your reader's attention.

Overall, very good work. With some careful editing, you'll have a winner.

Essay 84

I have exactly 5000 characters on this essay, I am just not sure where to cut down on. Thank you for your feedback.

As I took my first footsteps on Costa Rica, well known for its tropical beaches and thrilling adventures, I approached it differently than many other travelers did. I spent my vacation week at the National Children's Hospital in San José to discover more about the healthcare systems outside of the United States and to help those who are in need. Although Costa Rica is known for having one of the best healthcare systems in Latin America, I was still able to see the less developed parts. I met a 20 month-old baby boy admitted due to malnutrition. He had bright, intelligent eyes but was receiving treatments because he was not the normal size for his age group. That moment, when I saw people in pain so up close, was the moment when I determined once again to pursue a career in the field of healthcare.

I was always interested in pursuing a career in the healthcare field because I naturally find the human body system fascinating. I have considered other healthcare careers throughout my lifetime. However, I firmly believe that Physician Assistant (PA) meets all my criteria of having much patient interaction, ability to diagnose and prescribe.

After I had firmly decided to become a PA, I shadowed PA at the Endocrinology Consultants in Englewood, NJ. Having observed the physician assistants from the start of their day to the end of the day, I now understand the profession and the curriculum of a PA. I worked at a pediatrician's office for over a year as a medical assistant observing and learning closely from a doctor. In addition, I have volunteered at numerous hospitals both nationally and internationally. From those experiences, I learned that I love patient care and this is what I want to do for life.

I am a person of love and compassion. Because love is how I define myself, I have shown love to people who were unloved and because of my character, people naturally surrounds me. Ever since young I have been someone whom friends come for advice or for help when they are sick or are in need. I enjoy communicating and interacting with people, especially those who are in need of my help medically.

College was a turning point in my life where I discovered myself enjoying and working at my best when I work as a team. Since the beginning of time, humans could not live alone; we need each other and need to work together to bring the best outcome. In a novel The Great Wing, the author Louis A. Tartaglia tells a story of Canadian geese migrating for the season and how it reflects to human beings. The young geese hear about the "Flock Mind" ever since young and how to be receptive to the power of the Universe. Finally, the time for migration comes and Gomer, the protagonist, and his flock flies out strongly. They interchange the roles of leading the group and even the geese that seems to fail amongst the group does not founder from the "Great Wing" due to the help of other geese and eventually land at a new home for the season. As I read this book, I realized how similar it is to our human society. Unique individuals meet together to form a group and groups meet together to form a society. As a part of the society, we need to work together rather than fight for our own interest. Acknowledging the fact that we cannot live alone in this world leads us to live a life that is emphasized in the novel by Tartaglia. Thus, helping people in the world, medically, is also what I desire to do to contribute to the society that I live in.

Commentary Essay 84

Your compassion comes through loud and clear. Your patients will be lucky. Your opening is very good and only needs a bit of editing.

I would recommend cutting the description of "The Great Wing" and that fact that "you're a person of love," and focus more on the things that draw you to the PA profession apart from the need of people to work together and your love of patient care. There are a lot of other healthcare professions that have those qualities. What Admission's folks are interested in is what you bring to the profession and why it's right for you.

You say that college was when you learned you liked working as a team, but never flesh it out. You could tie those experiences to your health care experiences to show how it plays out for you. I'd rather see you write about that than spend almost an entire paragraph giving a synopsis of a book. Then add the rest of the information I've mentioned.

Essay 85

"I can't feel my arms..." were the first word's I heard my teammate scream after colliding heads with an opposing player. There were 10 minutes left in the championship game. One of our best players went head to head with another, and the next thing we knew was she was on the ground screaming. I immediately kneeled down and began to comfort her. I instinctually grabbed her neck to stabilize, and patiently waited for the crowding of coaches and parents. 911 was called and for the next what seemed like an eternity, waited for the ambulance to come. These 45 minutes were spent keeping Jackie calm as possible, yet also keeping myself cool as I was still holding her neck. The ambulance came, paramedics took over my role, and strapped her up into their van. One of them patted me on the back and told me I'd make a great doctor someday, and it was in that moment that I knew I belonged in the healthcare field.

Choosing what exactly I wanted to do with my life within the medical field did not come as easy as I hoped. I knew I loved sports, and I loved medicine, so I put the two together, and thought that going into athletic training was the perfect idea. I went through two years of an athletic training program, gaining more experience than I could have ever imagined. Working with Division I athletes and being a huge part of their successes was a wonderful feeling. Being able to capture the trust of athletes my own age was one of the most rewarding feelings in the world. I found I was driven by the constant feedback and follow up I was able to attain from each of my athletes. Day by day I was able to track where they progressed or lacked, making each athlete an ever-changing puzzle for me to solve. It was a hands on experience unlike any other I had encountered so far, but I knew I had more to discover. Working one on one with the athletes and coaches, and other athletic trainers was great, but what I enjoyed the most was working with the team doctors. They were the ones who ultimately got to take over the care of the injured athletes, and that was something I yearned to be a part of.

While the thought of medical school became a topic of interest, I felt like the job description was not entirely what I had in mind. I was introduced to a physician assistant, and suddenly it felt like everything clicked. Everything she had to say about the field, her job description, the pros and even the cons all sounded like exactly what I wanted to do. Shadowing her and seeing how a PA functioned within a hospital setting gave me the reassurance I needed. Having the ability to be more responsible for a patient's overall care and health became my biggest motivation. Kristin worked in what she called "fracture clinic." She evaluated patients injuries, sent them for x-rays or scans, diagnosed them, and even decided when to send them into surgery or not. While of course she worked under the care of a physician, Kristin was as in charge as she wanted to be. She had the option to treat the patient as she wanted, calling in for second opinions as needed, and every once and a while checking in with the doctor in charge. The gratitude she received by working with the patients and their families was really something that solidified that becoming a PA was the right decision for me.

I began working as a medical assistant for a pain management doctor. While I was a certified medical assistant, my knowledge and experience I had gained through the athletic training program would give me the basis of information needed to at least start in the position. My enthusiasm and willingness to learn new things, coupled with my positive attitude and aptitude to proactively take initiative paved the way for my successes as a medical assistant. Being one of two people that worked in the office, extreme multitasking became second nature and the ability to work in a fast paced, high pressure environment became a normality. Working in a small private office allowed us, even as medical assistants, to have the majority of the patient interaction. We were given the freedom to initially assess the patients, perform examinations, determine what we believed would be the correct treatment, and then follow up with the patients afterwards. This experience further convinced me that I was making the right choice.

I hope to continue my journey by becoming a physician assistant. I have come to appreciate the immense amount of time, patience, and critical thinking that goes into not only the years of schooling ahead but also my future in this profession. I look forward to my growth as a clinician and an active member in a field that is constantly expanding and advancing. When it comes to making the largest life decision thus far, it is the complexity and challenges presented within each and every patient that reassures me that I am making the right choice and investment for my future.

Commentary Essay 85

This is a really great essay. You cover all the important points, it flows well and you've made a convincing case for why you want to be a PA and why you'd be a very good one. Watch for grammar errors, though — you have a couple and they do matter to Admissions folks. When I interviewed Admissions Directors and faculty across the country about writing these essays for our book, "How To Write Your Physician Assistant Personal Statement," all said there shouldn't be any grammar errors, that it was a red flag that people didn't pay attention to details. In healthcare, missing the details can lead to death!

Essay 86

Every morning I am awakened by a vibrating noise accompanied by its disturbing ring that we all have suffered and dislike, but this particular morning was different. It was around 3 AM when I was awakened by this common vibrating and ring. My room was pitch black, except for the light shining from my cell phone as I was receiving a call from my mother. I knew for a fact, just like anyone else would, that something was wrong. My heart was racing, hands trembling, and my mind was thinking of the most horrible reasons for the phone call as I answered, "Hey mom what's wrong? Is everything ok?" She replied, "Your dad is in the hospital because he was experiencing chest pain and numbness." This immediately took me back to 9 years prior where my father suffered a severe car accident and was in the hospital for months with multiple injuries. I asked my mother, "Is he ok? What tests are they doing?" She replied, "Yes he's fine, don't worry. The doctors think he may have had a small heart attack, so they're doing blood work."

After spending the day in the emergency room, my father was released from the hospital with the diagnosis of acid reflux and indigestion. The doctor recommended that my father visit a cardiologist to be certain it wasn't his heart. My father followed the doctor's recommendation and the cardiologist had my father perform a treadmill stress test; in which the results came back normal. A month passed by and my father seemed to be doing better, until I received another early morning call from my mother about 5 AM and heard that my father was in the hospital again with the same symptoms. This time the doctors kept him overnight for observation, acquired more blood work, and ordered an echocardiogram. The results of the echocardiogram came back normal and his cardiac troponin levels were also normal; indicating that his heart had not been damaged. Once more, the doctors diagnosed him with acid reflux and indigestion and prescribed him medication to relieve his symptoms.

After this second incident, I was a bit skeptical about the doctor's diagnosis. I told my mother to watch him carefully when they sent him home because I had an uneasy feeling that something may happen again. Sure enough, I received a phone call that morning around 2 AM from my mother stating that my father was in severe pain. I spoke with him and he said to me, "Son you know that I can handle a lot of pain, but my whole entire stomach area is in excruciating pain and I don't know what to do. I have been to the hospital here twice and they haven't figured out what is wrong with me. I can't handle this pain, I feel like I'm dying." He was contemplating driving 70 miles to another hospital, but his pain was so bad that my mother took him to the emergency room at the same hospital. This time, he was greeted by a knowledgeable and compassionate PA who ordered morphine for my father's pain and listened to my father's symptoms. She ordered a stat ultrasound on his gallbladder and observed the ultrasound. She told my father that his gallbladder was full of gallstones and sludge, severely gangrenous, and it needed to be taken out immediately. Approximately 10 hours later, my father was out of surgery and in recovery. Today, he is doing awesome and we have been grateful towards the PA that saved his life.

So why do I want to be a PA? Well, this experience further enhanced my desire to become a PA because it helped me realize that not all doctors can determine the correct diagnosis and a PA is just as skilled as a doctor. The PA that helped my father found his problem in a matter of minutes whereas multiple doctors couldn't find the problem. She was very observant when he came into the emergency room and truly cared for his wellbeing. I could tell that she took care of every patient with the upmost respect and empathy in their difficult time of distress. This motivated me to further enhance my patient care skills and I am confident that by becoming a PA I will be able to improve these skills. PAs take pride in providing high-quality patient care to all persons no matter race, ethnicity, gender, social status, economic status, age, etc. and I am dedicated to learn new methods to improve this patient care and the lives of every patient that walks through my door. I strive to hear the words "Thank you for your help" knowing that I made a difference in a person's life and created a bond for the rest of my life.

Commentary Essay 86

Thank goodness your dad was lucky enough to find a good PA. I'm glad he's well.

The problem with the essay is that is basically all you talk about. You haven't mentioned anything about yourself and your experiences. Yes, your patient skills would improve if you became a PA. They would improve by doing a lot of different things.

Have you shadowed a PA? Spent any time working with them? If so, write about those experiences and why they helped form your decision to apply to PA school. Then talk about your own experiences, and what traits or skills you have that would be good for the profession.

I'm afraid that if you rely on the one experience as the reason you want to be a PA, it won't be enough. If that's all you have right now, do some shadowing or volunteer work to expand your knowledge of the profession and develop insights into yourself.

Consolidate the whole first part of your essay into a short paragraph. Then work on writing the things that will show admission's faculty you're a good candidate for the profession.

Let me give you an example of cutting. Here's what I would do with your first three sentences: At 3 a.m. my room was pitch black, except for the light shining from my cell phone signaling a call from my mother.

It may seem discouraging to have to change so much. But if you want readers to consider you, that's what you'll need to do.

Essay 87

My life journey of soccer began at age four. I played on my very first recreational team and continued to fall in love with the game that helped build my life to everything it is now. I could not wait to go to practice twice a week and show up for my games every weekend. As I grew older, I began to play soccer competitively, traveling across the United States almost every weekend. Soccer began to consume my entire life outside of school.

I was fortunate enough to not have any major injuries until my junior year of high school when I began to have problems with my knees and ankles. My injuries led to many appointments with the Sports Medicine doctor. My visits to the doctor sparked an interest with sports medicine and the medical field in general as I found it interesting to learn details about my injuries. My doctor was able to explain my injuries in full detail, which helped me understand and become more interested in what was occurring in my body. My senior year of high school I began to have issues with my feet which led to bunion surgery. As with my sports medicine doctor, my podiatrist explained, in full detail, exactly what my surgery was going to consist of and how my body would react, the recovery and subsequent rehabilitation to return to my sport. These experiences with my own injuries helped make my decision to pursue the medical field further.

Based on my interest to pursue the medical field for my career and specifically sports medicine, I begin to search for schools with outstanding Kinesiology programs. With the help of my athletic scholarship for soccer, and my high school GPA, I enrolled in the Fresno State Kinesiology Program: Exercise Science. As I played Division 1 soccer at Fresno State, my interest for the medical field continued to grow. As an athlete, I had a close relationship with the athletic trainers and the team doctors. Learning from them about the different injuries of athletes continued to stimulate my interests in sports medicine. While learning about the body and the science behind every system in our body, I became interested in Physician Assistant. The fascination of science aspects of our body made me realize that Physician Assistant for a career would be my ultimate goal. Physician Assistant will keep me engaged in the science and learning of the bodies anatomy and physiology along with gaining experience and knowledge of working with patients and other medical professions.

The time constraints of being a student athlete hindered my ability to get work experience in the medical field but I feel I was able to gain other exceptional skills as a collegiate athlete. After my last season ended, I was able to acquire an internship at the Saint Agnes Cardiac Rehabilitation Center. Although brief, my internship gave me experience in working with patients and gaining knowledge about the medical field. Being a student athlete taught me time management, multitasking, dedication, along with determination, hard work and being a team player. Learning how to manage my schoolwork while I was playing collegiate soccer became difficult at times. Learning to manage my time was a key component that helped me keep up my athletic performance while keeping my grades up. Knowing it was not an option to let my performance or grades slip, helped me push myself to the limit to make sure I stayed at the top in all aspects of my life. Dedication to my schooling and to my sport helped me continue my dream of becoming a Physician Assistant.

Dedication will become exponential in my journey to become a Physician Assistant because of the work that needs to be put into the program. Staying dedicated throughout the program will help fulfill the expectations of the program and the high demand placed on myself. My strong work ethic will assure that my work gets done in a timely manner and with the upmost quality of work.. Being a team player is key for Physician Assistant programs and in the work field. Working with others will ensure people are held accountable for their own success and the success of the entire class.

Helping others with their health, building relationships and continuing to gain knowledge about others will help fulfill my life with my dreams through becoming a Physician Assistant. I would be honored to enter a program and the work field of Physician Assistant to encourage quality work, compassion, hard work and adaptability to this amazing career.

Commentary Essay 87

You've done a great job of highlighting the strengths you've gained as a soccer player. Your dedication, perseverance, teamwork, time management are all excellent skills that will carry you far in your career.

You could cut quite a bit of your soccer experiences though, and should. For example, I'd edit the first paragraph like this: My life journey of soccer began at age four when I played on my very first recreational team. As I grew older, I played soccer competitively, traveling across the United States almost every weekend. I continued to fall in love with the game that helped build my life to everything it is now.

The way you refer to PAs sounds like you've just plugged it into a form essay. This sentence for example: Physician Assistant will keep me engaged in the science and learning of the bodies anatomy and physiology. Normally people would say becoming a Physician Assistant or the Physician Assistant profession. The way it's written you could substitute the word nurse or doctor or any other number of healthcare professions. By the way, don't capitalize physician assistant, and it's "body's anatomy," not "bodies anatomy." You want to make sure you do a careful grammar and spell check before submitting. Not every error gets caught, so have someone else proof your essay).

Which brings up the main problem — your essay suggests that you really don't know what a PA does. This sentence I quoted above is an example. There's no real tie to the job of PA other than a general interest in science aspects of our body. That's insufficient.

If you haven't shadowed a PA, you really need to spend some time doing it for two reasons. One, so you really know what the profession entails, and two, so you can communicate that in your essay. If you interacted with PAs in your internship, then write about it in detail. Even if your internship was brief, if you had contact with PAs make the most of it in your essay. That should make up the bulk of the essay, not your soccer experiences.

Essay 88

This is my essay from last year's cycle in which I was not accepted. I am looking to where I can better my essay.

"Jim, you need to settle down!" exclaimed the psychiatrist to the patient. Jim was suffering from Lewy Body Dementia. The first time I met Jim, he was delusional and unable to carry on a conversation. He was constantly trying to take his clothes off and throwing his food. The next week, when I returned to the Behavioral Health Unit (BHU), I was greeted by Jim with a huge smile on his face, sitting quietly in a recliner. Jim seemed like a different person. I met with the psychiatrists who worked with Jim numerous times throughout that summer. They taught me how they assess, diagnose, and treat patients like Jim to help them achieve lifelong wellbeing, a sense of normalcy, and freedom from their disease. The influence the psychiatrists from the BHU had on their patients was remarkable. Their patients were all in the end stage of their long lives, but the compassionate psychiatrists were able to help comfort their patients and the patients' families. It was this experience that inspired my desire to pursue a career as a Physician's Assistant. I want to provide support for those struggling with their health in unfortunate and unexpected situations.

Growing up in a small rural Minnesota community, life was simple, but I always wanted more in life. I left for college to broaden my perspectives. My first year at St. Thomas, I struggled being away from family and friends. I called my parents each night begging them to let me come home. My fear got the best of me, and my grades and potential friendships suffered. The next summer, I took an internship at Lakewood Health System. While working there, I was able to gain confidence and determination. I recognized my need to conquer fear. My time was spent in the nursing home and BHU visiting with residents, and shadowing providers. While observing the provider's interactions with patients, it was clear that health care requires a deep level of commitment and compassion for others. It was that same level of commitment and compassion I experienced growing up in a small rural community where relationships and individuals were valued. The relationships the providers built with their patients reaffirmed my desire to pursue a career in health care.

The next three years of college, I was determined to not let fear and my freshman year struggles impact my career aspirations so I created new challenges for myself. I established friendships and my grades soared. My junior year, I traveled half way around the world to study abroad in New Zealand. My time abroad gave me the passion to have, not only a well-rounded education, but a well-rounded perspective on life. I took nontraditional courses such as New Zealand Christianity and Forensic psychology. I was overwhelmed with the desire to learn new things, realizing that a well-rounded spectrum of knowledge was a necessity for success in life. I feel very fortunate to have the opportunities to pursue my life's passions. I want to help people who are suffering from illnesses that inhibit their ability to pursue their desires in life.

After shadowing numerous providers as a scribe and other internships, I knew medicine would be a rewarding profession where I could embark on a lifetime of learning; while providing a service to those in need. Though my first year in college was difficult, it was a necessary complication I needed in order to overcome fear. Through my determination, compassion, and desire for learning, I know I will be able to defeat any complication that arises when I am practicing medicine as a Physician's Assistant.

Commentary Essay 88

Good for you overcoming a huge barrier to your future success. It wasn't easy and you pushed yourself well beyond your comfort level. That will serve you well.

I see some issues with your essay. For one, and it's a big one, the profession is physician assistant, not Physician's Assistant. That is enough to make Admissions folks wonder if you just looked up careers on a website, and not a good website at that! It's enough to keep you from an interview.

Your essay can use quite a bit of editing. Overall, you can cut quite a bit from it to cover what is missing — why you chose the PA profession. You say you shadowed providers, but never mention any contact with PAs. Did you have any? If so, what about the work they did appeals to you? Apart from being a compassionate person, what personal strengths do you have that would make you a good PA? Admissions Directors and faculty need to know those things.

Less is going to be more in this essay when it comes to explaining your difficulties in your freshman year. Here's how I'd edit it:

"Growing up in a small rural Minnesota community, life was simple, but I always wanted more from life. I left for college to broaden my perspectives. My first year at St. Thomas, I struggled being away from family and friends and my grades and potential friendships suffered".

You want to approach your challenges from the most positive perspective you can so that people will see that you have the strength to overcome them. It's good to address poor grades, and you've done that. You just don't want to overdo it.

I rarely suggest professional editing for obvious reasons, even though most of the essays I review for free could greatly benefit from it. But since this is your second go-around, I would consider it to ensure you have the best essay possible.

Essay 89

I am a recent college grad applying to PA schools this summer.

Anxiously I approached a young pregnant woman dressed in traditional African attire, humming a soft lullaby to her sleeping son. Despite her tired eyes, her inviting smile somewhat eased my tension, as it was my first day as a patient advocate for Harlem Hospital OB/GYN clinic. I introduced myself and told her about our program. She concentrated on the flier for a few minutes before finally asking "what food?" I quickly realized she was unclear of what I just said, so I slowly and thoroughly explained how I can connect her to government subsidized benefits, food assistance, affordable healthcare options, or childcare resources for her son. After a few seconds, she finally leaned in closer told me that sometimes she worries she may not have enough money to provide a proper meal for her children.

I was in awe of the struggles she was already facing, considering she was only a few years older than me and already expecting a second child. We completed an assessment and I immediately got to work. My first priority was to connect her to the Supplemental Nutrition Assistance Program and the Women Infants and Children program, which provide financial assistance to low income families. Through weekly follow up calls and occasional visits, we made progress in navigating the application process. In the meantime, I gave her a listing of all the food pantries near her home, and informed her of the Early Head Start and Head Start child care programs for her son. Since she was unemployed, I also informed her about employment agencies that catered to non-citizens and people who had little to no education. I worked diligently to help her every way possible. The day she successfully enrolled in the SNAP program, she was very grateful and she called me."Thank you so much Sumaiya, I will call you if I need anything", she said. That was the last time I spoke to her, but the first time I knew that I wanted to continue to make such a difference for the rest of my life.

Through additional volunteer experiences in medical offices and hospitals, I gained insight into how health care professionals diagnose, treat, and prevent ailments of patients to ultimately promote a healthy life. The process of analyzing symptoms and administering treatment fascinated me, because it encompassed attention to a wide range of factors affecting the health of a patient. I observed Nurse Practitioners, Physicians, and Physician Assistants as they delivered patient care, and the role of a Physician Assistant appealed to me the most. There were two main reasons why I chose the PA route. First, I knew I wanted a career which followed the medical model; I wanted to be involved in determining the specific malfunction of the body and treating it. Second, I wanted the flexibility of exploring different specialties. If I work in Pediatrics for a few years and became interested in gynecology, I know I would have the ability to pursue that specialty seamlessly.

I further gravitated towards this career path, since the role of a PA resonated with my role as a patient advocate. As a patient advocate, I was able to discern other confounding factors that also played a role in the overall wellbeing of a patient. For instance, the financial stresses of a patient causing repeated visits to the doctor for complications due to high blood pressure, or the lack of proper knowledge and access to healthy eating habits adding on to complications with diabetes. As I occasionally shadowed a PA in the OB/GYN clinic, he educated me on the prevalence of alcohol abuse amongst pregnant mothers, which made their unborn children susceptible to a plethora of physical and mental disorders. I screened patients and connected them with the resources they needed, whether it was affordable health care, self-help programs, or food assistance programs to promote healthy eating. I also worked with my associate advocates and program managers every week to discuss issues with health disparities and ways we can further help our clients using the resources available to us in our city.

Up until that point in my life, I felt like I was living with my eyes closed. As I worked with the women of the OB/GYN clinic, I became more aware of the living conditions of the people of my city, and how multifaceted health care is. I opened my eyes to see that I was living in a city where people worried that they would lose their home because they could not afford rent, and teenage mothers struggled to provide their children with a proper upbringing. Working on these cases further instilled in me the importance of becoming a health care provider sensitive to the hurdles many patients experience living in underserved communities. To know I made even just a small difference to improve patient's lives as a Patient Advocate impacted me greatly. But more importantly I know I do not want to stop there. As a PA, I wish to provide my patients with optimal medical care and the knowledge they need to lead a healthy life.

Commentary Essay 89

You've done a lot for being a recent college grad. Congrats on that. You've gained great experience working with people living in poverty, and have great empathy for those who struggle. That will serve you well as a PA.

Before I forget, none of the following words are capitalized — Nurse Practitioners, Physicians, and Physician Assistants. You especially don't want to capitalize physician assistant. It's an instant red flag.

You could expand more on your experiences shadowing the PA and less about being a Patient Advocate. I'm not even sure from reading your essay why a career in medicine is for you. That's an important point. I was thinking the essay could be written for admission to a master's program in public health. Even though you're fresh out of college, you have to make a case for yourself why you'd be a good candidate for PA school. Healthcare, not social work is the foundation for the profession.

If you spend more time establishing the things I've talked about, you'll have an excellent essay.

Essay 90

I'm reapplying this year. Not sure if I should completely start over from scratch or if I should edit this one adding a few more current experiences.

"I feel like being a blonde today!" proclaimed my aunt as she prepared for her morning chemotherapy. Every session was another opportunity to not only reinvent herself, but also radiate cheerfulness to others enduring the same treatment. "Stop by Hot Cakes, please. I want to surprise everyone today." Whether it were fresh, moist cupcakes or personally knit beanies, she always conceived a way to spread contagious glee to others suffering. Despite her ailing health, she never lost her optimistic demeanor I grew to admire. She sees her cup as half full, and translates it into an opportunity to replenish the cups of others; a quality I have emulated throughout my pursuit to complete my ultimate goal: to provide superior healthcare to the less fortunate and underserved while fostering intimate and holistic relationships.

In 2009, my aunt was diagnosed with stage four breast cancer. Shortly after tests and referrals we were introduced to a Physician Assistant. My aunt's PA was the epitome of what I believe to be of a medical professional: eloquent, compassionate, patient and genuine. Through sincerity and amiability, she not only sub-sided our unsettling fears, but also prepared us for what was to come. Our lingering apprehensions soon dissipated and for the first time my family and I felt peace of mind. I truly valued and admired her bedside manner; she treated my aunt like family. She spoke directly to her despite me being her translator. Her empathy and genuine propensity to form a supportive relation-ship left a distinguishing impression and ultimately incited my interest in a career as a Physician Assistant.

God has provided several arenas of "good works" for us and He desires that we walk in them, fulfilling our purpose and calling. One arena in particular that has unequivocally impacted me is the community clinic I've been gratefully working with for the past three years. As a medical assistant, my duties vary, but the most fulfilling are my daily conversations with each patient. Without these invaluable interactions, I would have not been able to realize that to truly treat a patient's physical ailment, a healthcare professional must nurture both their emotional and spiritual needs. My time with patients is spent conversing, shar-ing the gospel, and learning about their individual personalities and backgrounds. Despite their afflictions, I witnessed that gen-uine interest, prayer and conversation are what patients yearn for; even a simple chat regarding how they perfected their me-ringue recipe can go a long way.

My experiences at the clinic have afforded me a great deal of hands on patient interaction and exposure to a wide range of ill-nesses, diagnoses, and treatments in the field of internal medicine. Specifically, I am learning about primary care, which is my intended field because of its comprehensive nature. Con-versing with patients, building relationships, taking vitals, assisting in various procedures, charting and collaborating with doctors and fellow medical assistants have only given me a small fraction of what I will be doing as a PA. These are elements that inspire and motivate me to continue pursuing a career as a PA and allow me to give back to the community in which I grew up.

Missionary work with Project Pueblo developed my passion for serving and solidified my growing aspirations to help those less fortunate on a global scale. Coming from an immigrant family, I viewed missionary work as an opportunity to give back and pay forward the blessings my family and I have received. Through Project Pueblo, I had the opportunity to witness medicine and compassionate care to the underserved Indian reservations in the Southwest. Though their possessions are meager, their appreciation for selfless acts is abundant. Even in an impoverished environment, hope can be attained through small acts of kindness. The Navajo Nation has not only opened my eyes to the suffering here in the United States, but also left lifelong impressions in my heart. Having the opportunity to serve an underprivileged and marginalized culture has humbled and enriched my perspective on the differing needs of different cultures, which will undoubtedly help me become a better serving Physician Assistant.

My blessings have allowed me opportunities to lead a fulfilled life, but to truly fulfill my life is to fulfill the lives of others. My experiences have helped me to mature and grow into a better serving individual. I am fully adept and have complete confidence that I will not only overcome the rigors your program will bring, but also see that I leave no single cup half empty. Similarly to my aunt, I see my cup as half full and I aim to share it with the world, and do my best to make sure every cup is boundlessly overflowing, globally and locally. Thank you for your time and consideration.

Commentary Essay 90

First, physician assistant is never capitalized unless it's part of a formal name.

I really like your aunt! What an amazing woman and great role model. I also like the way your essay opens. But we don't need all of the information in the first and second paragraphs. The same applies to your paragraph about missionary work. This sentence, for example, is redundant and general: "Even in an impoverished environment, hope can be attained through small acts of kindness." I always recommend that people leave out generalizations — this essay is supposed to be about you, the reasons you want to be a PA and what you bring to the table.

There are a number of other generalizations in your essay. They include the first sentence in your third paragraph about God providing arenas of "good works." Although I see that your faith is deeply important to you, many people feel uncomfortable with the topic. Unless the PA school you're applying to is one which envisions its graduates sharing the gospel with patients, I would omit the religious references from your essay.

Go through your essay and carefully cut anything that is general or redundant. That will give you room to write about what's missing here, specifically what has changed since you last applied. Every Admissions Director or faculty member I interviewed said that was critical. Tell what you've learned, how it changed you and better prepared you for the profession.

Here's how I'd edit the second paragraph:

"My aunt's PA was the epitome of what I believe to be of a medical professional: eloquent, compassionate, patient and genuine. She not only subsided our unsettling fears, but also prepared us for what was to come. I truly valued and admired her bedside manner — she spoke directly to my aunt despite me being her translator. Her empathy left a distinguishing impression, and she ultimately incited my interest in a career as a physician assistant."

Do the same with all your paragraphs, including the first.

Essay 91

Less than 3 minutes' left on the score board. Ball is just inside the 30-yard line. Quarterback takes the snap and throws a pass and gets blindsided by the linebacker. As I watch intently from the sideline, the quarterback lays lifeless on the turf and the referee blows the whistle. I run quickly out to the player on the field. He is alert but is obviously disoriented and is complaining of tinnitus and headache. The referee informs me the quarterback did lose consciousness briefly after the hit. After ruling out any other injuries I escort the player to the sideline treatment table. I took his helmet away and placed it with my medical kit behind the bench. I continue my sideline concussion evaluation. The player is in stable condition but he obviously cannot return to the field after suffering this injury. I turn slightly to motion to his dad in the bleachers to come down to the field and before I knew it my head coach had grabbed the quarterback and given him his helmet and pushed him back on the field and said "Go get'em." I tried to stop the game but the referees could not stop the game. I tried yelling at my head coach saying "He has a concussion and cannot play." The head coach just smiled, shrugged his shoulders and ran away. That was the point that I knew that PA school was definitely in my future. This was the moment solidified that my "desire for more" was definitely worth listening to.

I had always had a desire to go to PA school but I had a stable job as a Head Athletic Trainer and Adjunct Professor in the collegiate setting. In total, I spent seven years in college athletics and I enjoyed working with athletes thoroughly. I have had so many great experiences ranging from managing open fractures on the field to observing ACL reconstructions in the operating room to rehabbing athletes back to full participation from a devastating injury. These experiences made me a great Athletic Trainer and I looked forward to each and every day because I never knew what type of injury, illness or problem I would face. However, the "business of athletic s" often took healthcare decisions out of my hands many times which put my athletes at risk not to mention my professional liability.

That school year, 20112012, was my last year in the collegiate setting. Since that time, I have been working as an athletic trainer in what is called a physician extender role with a Primary Care Sports Medicine Physician. I have thoroughly enjoyed this experience. It has deepened my desire for "more." I spend a great deal of time evaluating injuries, documenting in EMR, administering balance and concussion testing, educating patients, casting and splinting factures, assisting in procedures in the office, communicating with school athletic trainers and a myriad of other tasks. Many people may say that I have found my dream job at my current setting, but I say I have found a catapult into my next level.

I plan to become a physician assistant, specializing in the area that I see fit as I go through my clinical rotations. Although I have a strong sports medicine and orthopedic background, I have found other specialties to be of interest as I have worked in primary care. I want to become a Physician Assistant so that I can continue to do what I love which is interacting with people, guiding and helping them. Just as I am a great Athletic Trainer I will be a phenomenal Physician Assistant because I have a great ability to connect with people and understand them in a way a healthcare provider needs to. I truly believe this is the right time in my life to pursue PA school. I may be older than the average

PA student but I the experiences I have had are priceless and will only be of advantage to me as pursue my dream career.

Commentary Essay 91

You have some really great experience, which gives you a big head start on your application. It gives you a great opening for your essay, too, until I got to the "lifeless" quarterback and found out he was alive. So just say "appeared lifeless" or "seemed lifeless."

That's a minor point, though. The biggest problem is that you spend half your essay talking about a career or working in a place where your opinion wasn't valued enough to follow your advice. At least that's the way it's written. It leaves a negative impression.

The point you want to make about being Head Athletic Trainer is the great experience you got. So skip all the details, meaning cut most of that first and second paragraph. You can conclude that section with the sentence starting, However, the business of athletics . . . The whole section on that part of your career should be about three to four sentences max. Don't conclude it with wanting to be a PA. You need to lay the groundwork first.

You say you always wanted to be a PA, but never say why. You say you wanted to do "more" (by the way, don't put that or "the business of athletics" in quotes), but that's essentially meaningless the way the essay is written.

After the second paragraph where you talk about your work as a physician extender, then you can say you want to be a PA. But you need to be specific. How did you come to this decision? What is it about the profession that appeals to you? Have you shadowed a PA or worked with one? If so, you can talk about those experiences and relate them to why you decided to apply to PA school.

Essay 92

I'm feeling stuck and just feel like I need some direction for this essay. I look forward to everyone's comments.

Life is made of checklists. Even before birth we are closely monitored to ensure that our bodies are developing according to the established milestones for health and development. Once we start school, more checklists of homework, projects, health, physical and character milestones must be reached before we can enter into society. Go to college, have a career, get married, have kids, be nice to others. Checklists are rewarding. There is nothing more satisfying than crossing something off a todo list and having tangible evidence of being a productive member of society that day. Unfortunately this mentality can cause us to miss the most important moments in life. I thought healthcare was about a means to an end but have discovered that it is really about changing people's lives.

I had only been on the job for about three weeks and it was one of my first solo days on the floor. I sat in my office and uncontrollably sobbed to my boss on the other end of the line. "I'm just so tired and we're leaving for our trip in two hours, I don't know if I can screen another baby" All I could think about was my checklist for the day and how uncomfortable and inexperienced I was. Seven babies, their parents exhausted from a night of no sleep and adrenaline pumping through their blood from the day before. Having already been in the parent's room once that morning with an unsuccessful outcome, fear flooded my system not wanting to inconvenience them. "Take deep breaths" Christina soothed, "leave the last one for tomorrow, they won't go home anyway. But you will need to screen one more before you go, you can do it, call me with any more questions." Putting the phone away, wiping the tears from my eyes and collecting all the courage and composure I could muster, I went back on the floor to get the job done.

Fast-forward a year to April 2015 to a Neonatal Intensive Care Unit suite. Mom and Dad had finished feeding Baby and were watching the mandatory video all parents must see before the screen begins. If all went well, Baby would finally go home, a brand new start for this family. The sensors started reading, the computer analyzed and I looked at the tiny human being cradled by Dad. Glancing up at the monitor it was clear that the baby would do well and my heart jumped at the thought of sending this family home with good news. I wondered if there were siblings at home to welcome Baby and what the future holds. Glancing at my own growing belly and wondering what our birth story would be like, I wheeled the equipment out of the room with a final "Congratulations!"

What I didn't know at the beginning of this long process of science classes, volunteering, new jobs and challenges was that book knowledge or shadowing experience are only a piece of the health care puzzle. Health care is not something you can check off your daily to-do list. In order for medicine to really be a part of health care, we must use our knowledge to touch the lives of human beings; to make a family whole after seeing their world fall apart. Although science and technology continue to advance, it is the human touch combined with masterful application of the science and technology that facilitate healing. Often, the hand of compassion is what encourages and gives confidence to the ill to own their healing process. That is why I will be a dedicated Physician's Assistant.

Commentary Essay 92

I was very engaged by the opening of your essay. Great theme and one I haven't seen before. But the second paragraph didn't really hit the mark. For one, I don't know how long ago this took place. More importantly, it didn't really show me much positive about you. I don't think you want to give the impression that when you're first starting a challenging new position that you dissolve in tears. I know that wasn't your intent, but that's what's on the page. The fast forward paragraph didn't solve the problem. The conclusion though, is good.

What's completely missing from your essay is why you want to be a PA. It sounds from reading it that you love your job and are good at it. The Admissions folks that are reading the essay will want to know what made you decide to become a PA.

Have you shadowed any? Worked with them? Write about those experiences. Write about the things that are different from the profession you're currently in that you feel would be more suited to your interests, personality and skills.

Essay 93

It has always been a joke in my family that I am a bit of a hypochondriac. With the onset of any abnormal symptom, I begin researching, intrigued by every new medical fact I come across, until I feel confident that I have solved my medical mystery. I ask myself, "what could this symptom mean?" and "what can I do to feel myself again?" The process is always the same. First I turn to Google for the more general responses. After narrowing down the potentials, I try to find the one that explains the majority of my symptoms and delve deeper into more reliable diagnostic research. Once I'm satisfied that I've found my answer, I explain to whomever is interested that I am either dying of some rare disease, or more likely I am suffering from some commonplace illness. Usually I get mocked, but even more often my diagnoses are actually correct. Friends and family members have started turning to me as their personal sleuth for medical advice, while simultaneously teasing me for the occasional obscure diagnosis. Whether they do this to get a kick out of my dedicated detective work, or to prepare me for my future as a physician assistant (PA) I do not know, but their encouragement instills me with confidence.

I have always had a passion for medicine, but more specifically for improving the quality of people's lives in a one-on-one way. All the work that I have done thus far in my life has always been about serving people. Though waitressing has been my longest job to date and isn't medically related I've never found the work meaningless. It reinforced what I already knew about myself— that I love interacting with a diverse variety of people from all walks of life. Having already had a background in customer service, I found it pleasantly surprising that being a patient care coordinator in a dermatology office was not so different than being a server in a restaurant. Each day I greet patients with a smile, ask them about their wellbeing, and then provide them with focused attention and quality care. Every patient I take into the examination room becomes my responsibility and my duty to tend to whether I am bandaging a postsurgical wound, clotting blood after a biopsy, or taking out sutures. The only difference is that I know when patients leave the office I didn't simply serve them a meal, I had a role in improving whatever ailment drove them to seek medical care. There is nothing more rewarding than the feeling of helping another person.

I didn't always know I wanted to be a PA, but sometime during my junior year of college I went to an informational session about the career that made it sound like such a perfect fit for me that I had to learn more about it. The ability to transition from one specialty to another without years of additional training appealed to me most. Though I am currently interested in general surgery, I'm also passionate about pediatrics and value the ability to seamlessly transition from one to the other. Since I personally see a PA, and am familiar with the role of a family practice PA, I decided to shadow a pediatric PA. She taught me some of the most ingenious tricks to get her restless, nonverbal patients cooperating. My favorite was when she would have the toddlers run up and down the hall so that she could appropriately evaluate their heart and lung function. I was in awe of her creativity and her ability to diagnose even the most noncompliant of children.

In addition to what I learned from shadowing, my admiration for PAs also stems from a personal experience. It was a PA who ultimately saved my father's life. He went to her with a bad cough, but with his history of smoking for over 20 years she decided to err on the side of caution and sent him for a chest x-ray. That's when they found the lesion in his lung. Because of her, he had a lobectomy that removed the stage 1A cancer that was growing inside him. She was able to catch what his physician did not based off such an insignificant symptom because she had the time to truly get to know him and remembered his history. I aspire to be a PA whose patients can say the same thing about me.

As a physician assistant, my focus would always be on the patient. I hope to catch the little details that could end up being lifesaving. My goal as a provider would not be to see the most patients, or produce the most profit for the company, but to dedicate myself to providing patients with the best possible care, and when appropriate, knowing when to transfer that care to someone with more expertise than myself.

Commentary Essay 93

Your essay really picks up after the first paragraph. Frankly, it won't impress anyone in the medical profession that you use the Internet to diagnose illnesses or that you're a bit of a hypochondriac. Some things are better left unsaid and those are two of them.

You could easily start your essay with the second paragraph. You could add more details about why the PA profession appeals to you. The ability to transition to other areas of specialty is not a particularly compelling reason to be a PA. There are so many more substantive aspects of the job that you could write about.

I'm concerned about your conclusion. It just drops off. Actually, I'd delete most of it:

As a physician assistant, my focus would always be on the patient, catching the little details that could end up being lifesaving. My goal as a provider would be to dedicate myself to providing patients with the best possible care.

If you want to add more, tie it back into your experiences.

Essay 94

Out of the fifty employees that I worked with, they chose me. It was a hot and humid Monday in mid-July, just like any other regular day at Luther Crest. At about high noon, a 15-year old camper was rushed to the emergency room after being smacked across the head with a paddle while paddle boarding with the other campers on the Waterama program. The Community Director, named Maddie, an Assistant Community Director, named Rose, and the bleeding camper drove the twenty-five miles into town in the rental 2014 Chevrolet Cruze. The camper was getting his stitches when Rose lifted up her shirt to show the doctor something peculiar; "Hey, are these chicken pox?" Without hesitation, or even a second glance, the doctor replied, "Yes, yes those are."

With stitches stitched and a newly diagnosed case of the chicken pox, the three of them headed twenty-five miles back to Luther Crest. The camper, enthused to be back at camp with his beloved camp friends and counselor, jolted out of the vehicle after it was parked. The Maddie and Rose's next task? Find me. That summer, I was a counselor as well as a day camp director. This particular week, I was a counselor on an onsite day camp, which meant that once the campers left site for the day around five o'clock, I was doing miscellaneous tasks like dishes, planning, and work projects.

"Rae Rae! We need to talk with you!" I turned around to see that Rose and Maddie had returned back from the emergency room a few hours after the incident with the paddle. I figured they wanted to talk with me about the gruesome, yet awesome, experience they had in the emergency room. But no, despite my curiosity and desire to hear about the bloody tale, I was informed that Rose had chicken pox and therefore could not be around the 150 young campers. After being told that I was the only one onsite that week that could handle what they were about to entrust me with, I was switched off of my onsite day camp and on to full-fledged leadership within seconds.

In fulfilling the leadership role at camp, my new duties were to attend staff meetings at 7:30 AM, lead Morning Movers and Alpha in the mornings, put together worships, pack Bible Study materials, facilitate All Camp Games, and lastly, fulfill the role of the nurse – in the absence of chickenpox, Rose and two other Assistant Community Directors. With all of these new tasks thrown at me, I was ready to take on the week ahead of me.

As it was my second summer at camp, I knew the ropes and what my general role was as an Assistant Community Director. I led activities and planned worships, among many other things, with ease. It wasn't until Wednesday afternoon that I ran into my first semi, not even, catastrophe. A counselor had come to find me while I was preparing for that evening's events to inform me that a camper named Isaiah, whose name has been changed for confidentiality, had stubbed his toe on a rock while down at the beach. I thought to myself, No big deal, I'll give the camper some ice and a Band-Aid. I headed over to the healthcare center to find a little boy sitting in a chair who was holding back tears, but clearly in pain. I talked with him about what had happened as I gathered the first aid kit and as I approached his injury, I saw that it was much worse than what I had anticipated. Now, this was not an emergency room-worthy injury, but it was an injury that involved more blood and detachments than a camp nurse was used to. Isaiah's big toe's toenail was hanging on by a thread as his toe bled. I knew he was in pain, and I continued asking him what his favorite part about the week had been so far, what his favorite meal had been, and other questions that distracted him from the fact that his toenail would be falling off sometime this week, if not later that night.

I stopped the bleeding, cleaned up the injury, and finally put a Band-Aid on him. He agreed to visit with me throughout the day so that I could change his bandaging. Throughout my first aiding, I felt that I created a bond with this camper. I was smiling to myself as I started to log his name and injury when I felt two little arms wrap around my waist. I looked down to see Isaiah's little self and huge smile smiling up at me and saying, "thank you." He quickly limped out of the healthcare center so as to soak up as much free time that he had left before I could even double check if he was alright.

This moment in my life was a pivotal moment for me. This moment is when I realized that I had a passion for helping people; more specifically, children.

The idea was simply a quick blurt in a list of postgrad options that my boss was spewing off to me. I had just finished talking with her about my worries and concerns for my life after graduation, as I had been struggling to find motivation to seek a career in my field. I was about to graduate from Concordia College with a degree in Dietetics, but the experience I had with dietetics was not the most positive and it did not involve enough human interaction; which did not flow well with my personality. I was dreading a life behind a computer screen writing menus and filing patient assessments on a computer. I asked my boss to go back a few options in her impromptu list of postgrad options for me. There was something that caught my attention more than any of the other possibilities she mentioned. That "something" was applying to graduate school to become a Physician Assistant. I thought about my passion for human service, and furthermore, I thought about all of the campers I have helped throughout my summers at Luther Crest; from homesickness to Isaiah's stubbed toe. The very idea of having a career based on making sure that every child is healthy made me smile from ear to ear. It was then that I decided that I wanted to pursue the opportunity presented before me: becoming the world's best Physician Assistant and helping all the children that come before me.

I have always been a people person, and am often described as someone who is personable and able to work with a wide variety of people. With the indubitable career satisfaction for myself, as well as the need for PAs, and the changes in healthcare, I believe that becoming a Physician Assistant will benefit me as well as the patients that I will come in contact with. For me, there could be nothing more rewarding than committing my life to the cause of bettering a child's.

Commentary Essay 94

It was fun to read about your camp experiences, but they aren't what will get you an interview for a PA program, which is your goal in writing this essay. I'd skip the camp experiences altogether, but it you want to use any part of it, reduce it to a couple of relevant sentences that are healthcare related.

There's no transition to the paragraph where you meet with your counselor, so you'll need to fix that. But assuming you create a transition, all of the sudden, you decide to be a PA when your counselor mentions the profession. Unfortunately, that's not compelling. Admissions folks want to know that you have experience with the profession, whether it's through shadowing, volunteering, work or even as a patient to ensure you know what the profession entails, and that it's the right one for you. They want to know specifically, what appeals to you about the profession and why, and not just from a description you read. If you don't have any hands on healthcare experience other than at Luther Crest, I urge you to gain some so you have credibility when you apply to a PA program.

Essay 95

She lay there still, lifeless as the priest delivered her Last Rights. Cancer had invaded her body, and her prognosis was grim. Her loved ones had gathered and anticipated goodbye. But then, miraculously, her health started improving. Each day brought her closer to a normal life, void of tumors. Her health care team defeated the odds and successfully cured her of cancer by utilizing aggressive treatments. I spent countless days next to her in her hospital bed, attempting to comfort her through the pain. We were not only cousins, but also dear friends.

Although I was young and unable to fully understand the circumstances at the time, nearly losing Allie had a profound effect on my life. I have her health care providers to thank for many of my favorite memories. Because of them, I have been able to watch Allie grow into the incredible young woman she is today. Because of them, I have had her companionship for the past 21 years. Because of them, I want to help families like mine.

Allie's cancer inspired me to dedicate my life to helping those in need. Along with participating in Relay for Life annually, I joined Dance Marathon, a fundraising organization for Children's Miracle Network. Through this organization, I witnessed miracles. I watched a child with severe hydrocephalus run and dance despite doctors predicting she would never walk. I played hide and seek and laser tag with a girl who has endured numerous heart surgeries in her short five years of life. Seeing these children so full of life despite their prognoses encouraged me to pursue a health care career.

In addition to participating in Dance Marathon, I started volunteering at the University of Minnesota Children's Hospital, where I became witness to more miracles. A premature infant, weighing just three pounds at birth, required constant attention. Her days were filled with uncertainties, and while her parents were at work, she would scream continuously. I spent hours holding her and relaxing her until she was discharged from the hospital after a grueling six-month stay. Comforting children like her through social interaction and watching their health improve until they are able to go home has fueled my fervor for health care. Every time I walk into the hospital to volunteer, I feel a rushing sense of belonging. I want to give new life to patients and their loved ones; I want to care for people during their darkest days and lead them to a future free from ailment. Each patient I have encountered has further solidified this decision.

I chose to follow this yearning to care for patients by working as a Certified Nursing Assistant. This is where I met Esther, an elderly woman on hospice care. Esther remains positive regardless of her diagnosis. She is selfless and caring, always asking about my day before I have the opportunity to ask about hers. Each time I enter Esther's room, she reaches out her hand, longing for companionship. I spend twenty minutes each night tucking her into her bed, applying lotion to her hands, and asking about her life. I have discovered that she is a devoted mother of six children and a former Navy nurse. Caring for Esther in her last months of life has been an incredibly rewarding experience. I have learned the importance of being an emotionally supportive caregiver. Additionally, I have been further inspired to become a health care professional.

While confident in my decision to pursue a health care career, I was formerly unsure which profession was right for me. Thus, I started researching careers and seeking advice from health care providers I was acquainted with. I shadowed a Dosimetrist, a

Clinical Lab Scientist, and a Registered Nurse. Though all intriguing, none of these occupations seemed to provide what I was looking for.

Accustomed to being a student leader, I was in pursuit of a career that promoted leadership. I wanted to share my compassion with patients of all ages and prescribe treatments to improve their overall wellbeing. After shadowing a Physician Assistant (PA), I knew I had found the right occupation for me. Kristine Gehrmann interacted with each of her patients with empathy and understanding. She genuinely cared about their emotional, spiritual, and physical wellbeing, and she displayed compassion unmatched by other clinician types; I have found this to be true, too, of other PAs I have met. Physician Assistants are outstanding leaders and considerate, devoted caregivers. With physicians as their mentors, they work as part of a team to reach goals and save lives. I found the career I had been searching for.

Leaving the clinic after shadowing Kristine, I encountered the same feeling of belonging I experience when I volunteer. I am confident in my decision to become a PA, and I am excited for a future dedicated to improving the lives of ailing individuals. I look forward to giving families more time with their loved ones, just as Allie's health care team did for my family.

Commentary Essay 95

I can tell you've spent a lot of time on your essay. I really like the opening and how you tied the conclusion to the it. Good job. It's fairly polished with one big exception. Never capitalize physician assistant unless it's in a name.

You could cut much of the Dance Marathon and volunteer work at the Children's Hospital info. The message is much the same and you don't need to go into so much detail. Just because you have 5,000 characters and spaces doesn't mean you need to use them all.

If you do want to add more, use the space to add details about your shadowing experience with the PA. Perhaps pick a specific patient to use as an example of things that you appreciate about the profession and why you're well suited to it.

Essay 96

Pain comes in all forms. The small ache, a bit of soreness, the random pain, and the normal pain we live with everyday. Then there's the kind of pain you can't ignore. A level of pain so great that it blocks everything out; makes the rest of your world fade away until all we can think about is how much we hurt.

This is the kind of pain that I saw in a young girl named Kristina. She trusted me enough to share her thoughts and her story with me. The thoughts in Kristina's head were "all I want to do is die, there's nothing to live for anymore", her bipolar disorder had consumed her thought process with words that no human being deserves. But she came to me. I had been working as a Psychiatric assistant for 6 months at a residential treatment center, and I had no idea the experience would change my life. I looked forward to every shift so I could talk to her and make her laugh, and maybe just for a minute give her mind a break from the daunting negative thoughts that controlled her. Not every day was good though. I remember on one particular day we were outside walking around the playground when Kristina spotted a piece of sharp metal laying on the ground. Kristina picked up the metal without hesitation, "I miss the feeling of having a razor in my hand, it's the only thing that really puts me at ease" she said. I allowed her to hold the metal in her hand while I talked to her about all the hard work she's done and the positive things in her life. Emotions were running high, she broke down crying, handed me back the sharp metal piece, and said "I really want to change; I think I'm ready to finally accept treatment".

She became especially fond of me after that day, because she said I reminded her of her big sister and that she could trust me with anything. Kristina continued to struggle with treatment and her controlling thoughts everyday and unfortunately after several baker acts she had to be sent to a different facility that could hopefully change her life for good.

The thing that really changed my life was the letter I received from her a couple of months later. Kristina thanked me for all that I had done for her and for supporting her throughout treatment no matter how difficult she had been. She wrote that she was in a much better place emotionally, and that filled me with overwhelming joy. I thought this is what I want to do for the rest of my life. In honor of Kristina and the countless number of patients that I've been able to help after her, I have been able to find a joy in my life like never before. I have been directly involved in healthcare for four years, and every experience has brought me great satisfaction. To be a part of a person's day is a wonderful blessing. Certainly, there are many pleasures in life. But, for me none is greater than that which we find in the healing touch of another.

Commentary Essay 96

Your essay shows you have great heart. But unfortunately, it doesn't show much else. The essay sounds like you're wonderful at your job and love it. In fact, you actually write, "I thought this is what I want to do for the rest of my life." (By the way, cut that line). So why apply to PA school?

You haven't said one word about that, and this is the essay that will teach Admissions Directors and faculty about you. They'll be happy you're a kind person who loves helping patients. That's not enough to make them want to interview you. They'll want to know why you've chosen the PA profession. What traits you have that will make you a good PA and what about the profession appeals to you.

If you haven't shadowed or worked with PAs, do so. If you have, write about those experiences and why the profession is one that suits you and vice-versa. You could easily shorten your writing about Kristina to one paragraph and move on to more relevant topics.

I'd do some line editing if I knew what you were adding, but since I don't know anything more about you, I don't think that will be helpful.

Essay 97

And the heart monitor rang, "beep beep beeep!" Time stood still as the squiggly lines flattened on the black, gaping screen. I was speechless, motionless, as the scene of my first patient death as a medical scribe settled. This frozen moment ended with a final thought – I want to save lives!

My passion for medicine began with, ironically, medical adversity. Years of unremitting abdominal pain, coupled with hospitalizations left me saying to myself, "enough is enough." First the ruptured appendix which led to the traumatizing septic shock, surgical interventions, and Crohn's subsequently. It was difficult to find a silver lining, however when I looked harder I found something even more precious. My toy stethoscope and syringe had always been my favorite toys as a child, but the ambition to provide medical care had not dawned on me until my own life encountered a patient's needs and sole dependency on health care providers. The empathy and compassion provided to me alongside the treatment stood out to me and defined my love for health care. Ever since, a sense of gratitude washed over me and pulled me to my passion of rescuing other patients who, like me, are imprisoned by disease and pain.

Volunteering at the emergency department exposed me to the world of medicine, more importantly, it helped me realize my dream career during my freshman year   physician assistant. Their profound knowledge and level of confidence as they practiced medicine independently captured my interest towards this profession.

Further disclosure of this occupation through shadowing experiences gave me a solid exposure and understanding of the duties entailed as PA. Working alongside physician assistants and physicians gave me good synopsis of the two professions. The attendings I worked with spent most of their time supervising overall flow and management of ED patients, which is imperative, but my primary interest lies within the concept of personally being able to treat patients, often obtained through maximal patient contact. I noticed PAs were able to provide intricate quality care by spending an extended one on one time with patients.

Aside from fully manifesting my dream, through patient contact experience, medical scribing

helped me build close relationships with talented physicians, who as my mentors, challenged me to take a step further. In light of this together with my self determined and highly motivated nature, I decided to pursue medicine. Going back to school to complete the additional med school prerequirements served as a blessing in disguise. Balancing time between school and my demanding occupation, although challenging, showed my ability to multitask in a resilient manner. More so, my upward GPA trend reflected my determination and maturity as a student, thus preparing me for the rigorous coursework PA schools offer.

At the back of my mind, time had always been a crucial factor for me, to secure a stable career. Being the only family member present in the vicinity, I felt obligated to take up the responsibility to support my parents as they are approaching their 70 mark. This time crunch led me back to my first love Physician Assistant.

More so, the sincere compassion and empathy each PA displayed as they offered undivided time and attention towards their patients reminded me of my personal experience. This stood out to me the most and reopened my eyes that PA is the most promising career for me. Although my heart lies in emergency/critical care medicine but the ability to switch between specialities is definitely a plus.

Witnessing the tragedy and triumph of the ED escalated my interest and fascination for medicine. The determination of the physicians as they attended to critically ill patients touched my heart the most. A case I will always remember was an unresponsive autistic patient that was rushed in after a fall. His blood oxygen saturation level drastically fell to the low 60s, requiring an emergent intubation. The procedure anomalously took thirty minutes due to the abnormal development of internal organs in the patient, as noted by my doctor. My heart raced silently while my fingers became clammy with distress. Finally the trauma PA miraculously placed a chest tube and the patient was declared stable, giving me a sigh of relief. Picturing myself in that situation, affirmed my aspiration I want to be like that!

In addition to amplification of my love and respect for this field, the knowledge I received has helped me cultivate essential skills communally present among these providers. For an instance like: getting a head start on the transfer protocol for a patient suffering from acute 3rd and 4th degree burn injuries, while the doctor was busy stabilizing the patient, or analyzing and selecting the most reliable imaging study and view for a correct diagnosis.

Critical thinking and communication skills were a few of the skills I was able to refine, initially acquired while serving as community service chair of my greek organization. This role helped me encounter eye opening experiences that unveiled the reality of pain and suffering people undergo. The most memorable moment was retrieving a smile from a blind patient for simply feeding her a thanksgiving meal.

Just like the force of magnets, similarly, healthcare has tremendously impacted my life to the point that I cannot imagine myself doing anything else apart from this.

Like detours, life takes unexpected turns but will surely bring us to our final destination. Learning to embrace this journey was a challenge, but now I have never been more persuaded to pursue this career path have chosen, my first love, Physician Assistant.

Commentary Essay 97

I suspected when reading your essay that it was significantly over the word count just by looking at it. The kind of editing it could really use is more than I can do in this setting. But you can cut down by remembering your job in this essay is to convince Admissions Directors and faculty that you understand what the profession entails, why it's the right one for you and why you're right for the profession. It's hard to edit our own work — I know that from personal experience. So if you can't afford a professional edit, have people in the medical field, preferably PAs review it.

Here's how I would edit your second paragraph: My passion for medicine began with medical adversity. Years of unremitting abdominal pain, coupled with hospitalizations left me saying to myself, "enough is enough." It was difficult to find a silver lining, however when I looked harder I found something even more precious. The empathy, compassion and treatment provided me led me to pursue a career in health care.

You can see how this keeps your paragraph concise and focused. This is the kind of careful cutting you'll need to do. Skip the big words and keep it simple.

By the way, physician assistant is not capitalized unless it's in the name.

Essay 98

"Time of death, 7:59 AM." I clearly remember the time because every morning at 8 AM, the little boy in bed would beg his parents to let him watch SpongeBob. Immediately after his heart failed, the room was silent, save for the flat line from the heart monitor, and the opening theme song from SpongeBob. That little boy, Carlos, was one of my first patients when I started working as a phlebotomist at Robert Wood Johnson University Hospital. Carlos had been diagnosed with acute lymphoblastic leukemia; he had been given a good prognosis, and was being administered chemotherapy. For a while, Carlos seemed to be doing better, and then unexpectedly he took a turn for the worse. That morning, I walked into the room ready for the usual blood draw; I was fully expecting to see him at the edge of his bed, ready to sing along, and instead I saw him for the last time.

It was my first experience that uncertainty is just as prevalent in medicine as it is in life, and it was a jarring experience that stuck with me. I come from a traditional Guyanese background with a large close-knit, extended family which has been my support system for as long as I can remember. The month before I began my freshman year in college, my sister ran away from home. The aftermath left my family torn apart, and before I could even fathom the reality of the situation, my entire support system had been ripped to shreds. For a long time, I refused to accept that my family foundation had crumbled, and the struggle resulted in both academic and social distress. Since then I have come a long way, I have learned how to deal with the obstacles that crop up in life; I have learned to not get bogged down by the negatives, and to see the positive aspects of every situation.

When Carlos passed away, I was taken aback, disheartened, and given a dose of medical reality; it took effort, but I focused on the positives. Acute lymphoblastic leukemia has a 90% survival rate, but there is no way of knowing if your patient will be in the 10%. I took solace in knowing that the team treating Carlos had done absolutely everything they could, exhausted every treatment option, and tried to make him feel as comfortable as possible. I never imagined a situation like this as a little girl with aspirations of being physician assistant. I grew up with a natural affinity for science, it fascinated me and I couldn't get enough. From the anatomy of the tiniest ant to the complexity of the human body, it was all enchanting. As a young girl, my curiosity for science naïvely ignored the harsh truths of medicine. As a young woman however, I understand the uncertainty, and the loss of life; which makes me truly appreciate the opportunity to work tirelessly to make a huge difference in someone's life.

Throughout my experiences of shadowing, volunteering, and working in doctor's offices and hospitals, I have gotten a small understanding of how it feels to make an impact. There have been times when no one has been able to find a vein on a critical patient, and I was the only one able to draw blood from them. I have also had the opportunity to closely monitor patients over the course of a few years, and see them overcome serious health problems and grow to lead healthy lives. These moments and experiences have developed into an insatiable thirst to impact as many lives as I possibly can. These moments and experiences motivate me to go to PA school, motivate me to become a physician assistant, and motivate me to see the positive in every situation.

Commentary Essay 98

You have an excellent foundation for your essay. The opening story about Carlos is heartbreaking and real. You're a very good writer, and the essay flows well.

I don't know if your essay got posted in the format you intended, but you need a new paragraph starting with "I come from a traditional Guyanese background. . . " Then you need another new paragraph when you go back to Carlos.

You come close to telling why you want to be a PA, but don't quite get there. You need a little bit more to let Admissions Directors and faculty know why you're choosing the PA profession over all the other professions you came in contact with when you shadowed.

There are lots of places to cut. For example, you could rewrite this paragraph as follows:

I come from a traditional Guyanese background with a large close-knit, extended family which has been my support system for as long as I can remember. The month before I began my freshman year in college, my sister ran away from home. The aftermath left my family torn apart, my entire support system ripped to shreds and I suffered both academic and social distress.

The same is possible with other paragraphs, too, to leave yourself some space to add a little more information.

Overall, it's well done. With some careful editing and the addition of a little more information, this will be a great essay.

Essay 99

At the age of ten, I knew very little about cancer until my dad woke one morning with severe chest pain. After many tests and several days in the hospital, a biopsy of a lymph node confirmed it to be Stage II Hodgkin's Lymphoma. At the time I didn't realize exactly what this meant, but from what my mom, an oncology nurse, had told me – it wasn't good. During the following months I watched my mom care for my dad through the pain, nausea, and fatigue that come with chemotherapy and radiation. I even remember her telling me and my sister not to touch the Neulasta syringes in the fridge because "They're worth a lot more than the fridge." As I watched my mom care for my dad, I was fascinated by how she could start IVs, give shots, and generally make people feel better. I especially loved when she took me with her to work and I could watch her treat patients in an outpatient clinic. However, as I grew older my curiosity about medicine increased, and I wanted to know more about how medicine worked and how the body responds to it.

During this time, I went to Mexico on a weeklong mission trip. One afternoon after an event, a man with broken English invited a few of us to his home in order to pray for a sick family member. Inside his house of scrap metal and plywood we found a young, thin woman in obvious pain who we discovered was dying of bone cancer. We prayed and spoke with the family awhile, but as we left I couldn't help but compare the family with my own. This woman dying of cancer could have been my dad if we had not had access to medical care. Although brief, this encounter sparked my desire to not only pursue a career in medicine, but to care for the underserved as well.

Soon after the trip, I learned of the physician assistant profession through a family member. Its rigorous academics, opportunity to switch between specialties, and emphasis on serving the underserved were especially appealing to me – not to mention the ability to practice medicine with two and a half years of graduate study. My expectations were reaffirmed when I shadowed a physician assistant working in oncology. Not only was she extremely knowledgeable about her specialty, she was also very compassionate and put her patients at ease, all while maintaining a professional demeanor. Before shadowing I had considered both nursing and medical school, but as I watched her my decision to become a physician assistant was confirmed: it satisfied my desire to be challenged intellectually, to serve others, and to be able to do both within the next few years.

As a student looking forward to becoming a physician assistant, I have enjoyed learning the science behind medicine, especially when I can make connections with my clinical experience. For example, while studying hemoglobin in my biochemistry class, I transported and cared for a girl with sickle cell anemia and had a more thorough understanding of the EMT protocol because of this. I also regularly utilize my Spanish classes, especially Spanish for Healthcare, in order to help me communicate with the Hispanic patients and families that I encounter in EMS.

Since my dad's recovery from Hodgkin's, I have learned much more about Hodgkin's lymphoma other than it's "bad" and requires expensive shots. Learning about Reed Sternberg cells, how cancer is staged, and how to conduct a physical exam in Spanish have strengthened my anticipation for what lies ahead – particularly for working with Hispanic or rural communities as a physician assistant in either primary care or oncology. With my past experiences and future goals in mind, I hope to continue my journey in medicine and maybe even restore life to someone else's dad someday.

Commentary Essay 99

I was very glad to read your dad recovered from Hodgkin's. That was the first thing I looked for in the essay. In fact, I skipped the rest of it until I found it. I'm afraid Admissions folks who read your essay might do that, too. Tell us up front

You have a lot of good information in the essay, but it's disjointed. It didn't read well when you start with a very serious incident — your dad has cancer, and then switches to how you loved to go with your mom to her work. Then it moves to this: "However, as I grew older my curiosity about medicine increased, and I wanted to know more about how medicine worked and how the body responds to it. During this time, I went to Mexico on a week-long mission trip."

The entire first part of the essay is missing transitions, to take the reader from one thought and scene to the next. That being said, the second half of your essay is more cohesive and you did a very good job of explaining why you chose to be a PA over any other profession. I like your conclusion, too — it relates back to your opening.

Rewrite the first part and you'll be in good shape.

Essay 100

Helplessness and frustration. Those are the two main feelings I've experienced as an EMT. These are the feelings I have felt when I knew there was something more that could have been done for my patient, but was restricted by my scope of practice and knowledge, thus disabling me from providing that higher level of care that my patient would have benefited from. In my time as an EMT, I have had many different patients ranging from end of life care, where I literally could not do anything for them in my time with them, to patients being discharged from hospitals completely healed. They all mattered to me; they all helped shaped me into becoming better person and EMT. However only a handful of them have had such an impact that I remember every detail of the call and how I could have done more for them if only I knew how.

I had transported Patient X several times before this day, the last time being just two days prior. That last time I noted that her urine in her Foley catheter bag was a darker color than it usual was. I pointed it out to her and told her to keep drinking her water just as she'd been doing and left. I came back two days later to transport her to one of her last radiation appointments. I checked her Foley catheter bag again, this time the urine was cloudy and the air around her had that distinct smell that I had smelled before with patients' with a urinary tract infection. I looked at my partner and could tell he was thinking the same thing. We continued on with our transport and noticed her vitals were slightly elevated than normal which contributed to our suspicions of a UTI. We sat through her appointment and listened to her husband complain how their social worker wasn't helping them out in getting a nurse to help them out at home with his wife's care and how he had to be there with the caregiver they currently had for her to do anything regarding his wife's care. We realized then that we would have to speak up and advocate for this family for them to get the help they needed. We asked our dispatcher, who also happened to be a nurse, what our options were regarding the UTI that we were sure our patient had. We were told since she wasn't in any immediate danger from the infection, meaning the infection wasn't serious enough, we had to leave it up to them if they wanted to go to the ER or not. They decided to go back home to hear what their social worker had to say. After arriving back home and positioning her back in bed, I decided to delay us and wait until the social worker arrived. She came and when I told her the family's concerns for a nurse and medication pickups, I could tell she heard it before and didn't feel it necessary to hear it again. Then I told her my suspicions of Patient X having a UTI, made my findings and reasoning clear as to why I thought she should go to the ER. Again, I was brushed off and told that she'd look into it. After all, to her, I was "just an EMT".

To me, even if I was wrong about the UTI, I felt it necessary this patient should have still been given the opportunity to be checked out. I felt that if the infection really was a UTI and it became worse without treatment, all the progress she had made with her cancer, had the possibility to be undone in her weakened state. As I walked out of Patient X's house she and her husband looked at me with a small smile, almost like they was showing their gratitude to me for what I had tried to do for them. As little as I thought it had done, it made a huge difference to them personally having someone try and stand up for what Patient X needed. As I walked to the ambulance with my partner, he could tell how upset I was with the situation. He turned to me and said, "We're in the business of taking people to be fixed by other people. We're not the ones that do the fixing." I don't know if that statement was to make me feel better for doing as much as I could for Patient X and being brushed off for it, but that was the exact moment that I had realized that I needed to be on the other side. I needed to gain the skills and knowledge to be the one 'doing the fixing'. That was the exact moment I knew I needed to become a Physician's Assistant.

I have always wanted to make a difference in people's lives and I've tried to through my various experiences as a volunteer and EMT, but that was the moment I knew that I really wanted to be the person they trust enough to come to and allow me find the cause of their health issues and help them get better. That was the moment I knew, if I had the higher scope of practice and increased knowledge, I would do my absolute best to ensure patients received the best possible treatment.

Commentary Essay 100

You have an unusual approach in your essay, and it caught my attention. One thing that really caught my attention is that you got the name of the profession wrong. It's not "Physician's Assistant," it's 'physician assistant. Every Admissions Director I interviewed said that was a big red flag — it made them wonder if the person knew anything about the profession.

There are some things I'd cut so it's not quite as negative sounding, like "where I literally could not do anything for them in my time with them." Read your essay carefully and look for those negative statements that might be misconstrued.

One problem for me is that I'm not sure how being a PA would have changed anything for Patient X. I understand that she's the patient who made you decide you needed be on the fixin' side. It's not the best example, though.

You'll need to write why you decided to become a PA as opposed to any other healthcare provider. Why not be a doctor? You can cut quite a bit of what you wrote about Patient X. Here's an example of a few edited sentences:

We were told since she wasn't in any immediate danger from the infection we had to leave it up to them if they wanted to go to the ER. They decided to go back home to hear what their social worker had to say. After arriving back home and positioning her in bed, I decided to wait until the social worker arrived. She came and when I told her about the family's concerns and my suspicions about the UTI, I was brushed off and told that she'd look into it.

Essay 101

"Stop screen cheating," was a common phrase in my basement, usually followed by choice words. In between two a day football practices my friends and I would play Call of Duty. We were focused on playing sports and having fun, but we were full of youthful ignorance and self absorption. I tried my best to fit in with the stereotypical jock crowd, but my curiosity, passion for learning, and association with different groups of people, sometimes made me feel like an outsider. My effort was not focused solely on sports, like many of my peers, but on finding a meaningful career choice and excelling as a student athlete. Fortunately, I was able to interact and learn from many different people in my life. These experiences have taught me how to embrace challenges, using them to mold myself into an empathetic caregiver, educator, and communicator, all of which will serve me well in the collaborative role of a Physician Assistant.

Perhaps my biggest fan, and the person who provided me the most pivotal life experience, was my grandpa. He went to all of my sporting events, even when he couldn't remember which number I wore. My grandfather was influential in building a sense of community in my town of 7,000. Having owned a shoe store on Main Street for 30 years he was something of a celebrity in my town. I always respected how he treated people, oftentimes cutting deals for families so their children could have new shoes for school. He always preached to, "Kill them with kindness." At my games people would come up to shake his hand, but he wouldn't recognize them. He was degrading in his struggle with Alzheimer's, which would lead him into our home, as he needed full time care. My first foray into caregiving was a joint effort between my mother, a RN, and me. Taking care of my grandpa caused me to reevaluate my priorities, and work toward doing something to add value to the community. He taught me the value of compassion. When I look at a patient today I don't try to "kill them with kindness," but I do treat them as if they were my grandpa.

Much like a team working in unison, the body relies on many moving parts to maintain homeostasis, if one of these parts doesn't do its job, the entire system breaks down. While course-work taught me how to explain the inner workings of the body, nothing was as influential in giving me an understanding of how a small change can affect the entire person, quite like my Uncle Brad. During college I witnessed my Uncle losing his battle with Bipolar disorder. He would call to talk about my games, but his calls were filled with manic delusions. The tragedy of my Uncle's life helped me to connect the breakdown of the body with the overall human experience. His inability to function as a father and a member of society showed to me the importance of early detection and proper care. If we are able to educate our patients on how to maintain their wellbeing it will positively impact not only them and their families, but society in general. My Uncle showed me that we are all part of this team, and healthcare provides the means to repair and maintain the physical and mental health of each piece.

Unfortunately, each patient one deals with is not a relative or an adoring fan. Working as a Patient Care Assistant at Mayo Clinic I have witnessed the frustrations of providing care for confused or uncooperative patients. My times with these patients have shown me the importance of communication and establishing trust between patient and provider. For instance, while caring for an elderly destitute Cambodian woman, my job was to famil-iarize her to her surroundings, a difficult task with her inability to understand English. Despite the efforts of a translator, she refused to cooperate with the medical team. Over the course of the day I showed her around the hospital, where she marveled at all of the commotion. Later on I could tell by her body language that she was in distress, something that I pick up on due to my mild hearing loss forcing me to directly focus on the patient. She broke down weeping. I took her hand to let her know not every-one had abandoned her. At the end of the day she gave me a big bear hug, a hilarious sight according to my coworkers as I towered over her. Being able to impact her and get her to cooperate with the medical team solely through nonverbal communication helped solidify my decision to pursue the PA profession.

In truth I am very much a jock. I still miss the camaraderie of teammates, the grueling five a.m. lifting sessions, and the thrill of victory. Perhaps the greatest part of a team is working as a unified group toward a common goal. I don't think the jump from a sports goal to the goal of patient wellness is that far. Each situation is challenging, each victory relies on cooperation, and every goal is only obtained when one goes beyond the call of duty because of how much they care. Being a care provider isn't always easy, but as I have learned achieving a difficult goal makes it all the more special.

Commentary Essay 101

This is a very engaging and well done essay with a few minor problems (you're slightly over the character/space count and capitalized uncle throughout — it's never capitalized unless part of a name, "Uncle Brad"), and one larger one. The larger one — while you deftly list many aspects of the profession with your compelling family/patient examples, many of those things are common to other healthcare professions. You'll want to tie those to the PA profession more carefully. It won't take much — a few words here and there (which I believe you're capable of doing from your writing ability) will do the trick. You'll have to cut a few words to do this, but it will be worth it in the end to truly have an essay that answers the call of the question, "Why I want to be a physician assistant."

Final Thoughts

I hope these personal statements left you inspired and eager to start your own.

These essays are just a fraction of the many we receive through our PA school essay collaborative. The collaborative is a place where you can ask for free advice or find more personalized help through our editing service. Our editing services include one-time edits and one-on-one work sessions. We're here to help, with services tailored to your needs and budget. Learn more about what we offer at www.thepaessay.com.

I truly believe that each and every one of you reading this book has a gift to offer the world. There is nearly an infinite well of healing and human kindness inside of you. Success (and happiness) usually comes when we stop thinking about how the world affects us, and instead focus on how we can affect others.

This is what I experience every time I go to Haiti on medical mission trips. It is there, in the battered and torn dirt streets, amid the smell of burning trash and human excrement, bathed in the smiles and the sounds of children's laughter, giving medicine for free without an expectation for anything in return, that I feel most human. It is also the culmination of why I believe we all choose a career in medicine.

My belief is that it is in this place where you will find the words to paint your essay. Whether those feelings come from a medical mission trip or helping a patient at your local clinic, this is the place of humanity where we all can say, "Yes! I get it."

Now it is your turn.

It is your turn to stop making excuses and start making progress towards your goals.

We look forward to learning your personal journey and helping you reach your dream of joining the PA profession. You'll find us at www.thepalife.com

Warmly,

Stephen Pasquini PA-C

ABOUT THE AUTHORS

Stephen Pasquini PA-C

Stephen has been a physician assistant since 2004 and creator of www.thepalife.com. He is a National Health Service Corps Scholar and graduate from The University of Medicine and Dentistry of NJ (Rutgers) PA program and the University of Washington in Seattle, WA. Stephen has been working as a mentor and adviser to PA students through his website and personal practice for over 14 years. His passion is helping people express a gift for medicine and healing through the PA profession. His goal is to help compassionate, caring and patient-focused individuals actualize their dream of becoming a physician assistant.

Sue Edmondson

Sue Edmondson is the editor in chief at the PA Life Personal Statement Collaborative. She has helped hundreds of aspiring PA students edit and revise their personal statements through our free and paid service with unbelievable success. Sue is an award winning freelance writer who has written in Northern Nevada and Northern California since 1999. Her articles have appeared in magazines such as Edible Reno-Tahoe, Reno Magazine, reno.com, Enjoy, Family Pulse and RLife, and the Reno Gazette Journal and Mountain Echo newspapers. She dabbles in fiction, has sold several children's short stories and was awarded first place for short fiction by the Reno News and Review. She is co-author of "How to Write Your Physician Assistant Personal Statement," for which she interviewed Admissions Directors and faculty from top physician assistant programs across the country. Her other career is as an attorney and judicial officer. After spending several years practicing family law, she spent the next

19 years at the District Attorney's Office before serving as a family court master for eight years.

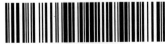

Made in the USA
San Bernardino, CA
06 December 2017